Drug Abuse Treatment

Drug and Alcohol Abuse Reviews

Edited by

Ronald R. Watson

- **Drug Abuse Treatment,** *1992*
- **Alcohol Abuse Treatment,** *1992*
- **Liver Pathology and Alcohol,** *1991*
- **Drug and Alcohol Abuse Prevention,** *1990*

Drug Abuse Treatment

Edited by

Ronald R. Watson

University of Arizona, Tucson, Arizona

Humana Press • Totowa, New Jersey

999 Riverview Drive
Totowa, NJ 07512

 9 8 7 6 5 4 3 2 1

Printed in the United States of America.

Library of Congress Cataloging-in-Publication Data

Drug abuse treatment / edited by Ronald R. Watson.
p. cm. — (Drug and alcohol abuse reviews)
Includes index.
ISBN 0-89603-233-7
1. Alcoholism—Treatment. 2. Drug abuse—Treatment. I. Watson, Ronald R. (Ronald Ross) II. Series
[DNLM: 1. Drug Treatment Centers—organization & administration—United States. 2. Substance abuse—therapy. WM 270 D793432]
RC565.D74 1992
616.86'06—dc20
DNLM/DLC
for Library of Congress 92-1691
CIP

Contents

Preface

A major national goal is to improve the health of the populace while advancing our opportunities to pursue happiness. Simultaneously, there are both increasing health costs and increasing demands that more be accomplished with less financial support. With the number of deaths attributable to drug abuse, especially of tobacco, in the US at about 250,000 per year, the annual cost of drug addiction is over $150 billion. Improved treatment methods can both reduce these costs and improve health by preventing the continued exposure of abusers to the toxic effects of alcohol and other drugs. This fourth volume of *Drug and Alcohol Abuse Reviews* focuses on the strategies currently thought best for the treatment of drugs of abuse.

A variety of approaches to drug abuse treatment employ those psychosocial factors that are known to influence drug use in youth and adults. Although the main emphasis is on the treatment of illicit drug use, a major cofactor in damaging the health of drug users is nicotine (tobacco) addiction, whose treatment is also reviewed. And the roles of learning and outpatient services are shown to affect treatment significantly. Thus, the problems confronted and solutions used in drug abuse treatment have here been analyzed in concise reviews that deal with the evidence for today's best hypotheses and conclusions. Some emphasis is also placed on reviewing new compounds used to prevent cocaine and opioid dependence.

With a wide range of such treatment options, many only partially tested, it becomes critical to evaluate and choose the most effective therapeutic systems for a given population. The present collection of critical survey articles constitutes a thorough examination of the issues and strategies particularly associated with treatment regimes for nicotine and other drugs of abuse. Since this volume brings together concise, definitive reviews of treatment and suggests ways to improve them, it will, one hopes, prove exceedingly helpful in understanding and planning what still remains to be done.

Ronald R. Watson

Contributors

Thomas G. Aigner • *Laboratory of Neuropsychology, National Institute of Mental Health, Bethesda, MD*

M. Douglas Anglin • *Drug Abuse Research Group, Neuropsychiatric Institute, University of California, Los Angeles, CA*

Thomas A. D'Aunno • *University of Michigan, Institute for Social Research, Ann Arbor, MI*

Yih-Ing Hser • *Drug Abuse Research Group, Neuropsychiatric Institute, University of California, Los Angeles, CA*

Anne M. Joseph • *University of Minnesota, Minneapolis, MN*

James M. Kaple • *Division of Applied Research, National Institute on Drug Abuse*

Thomas R. Kosten • *Connecticut Mental Health Center, New Haven, CT*

Robert M. Post • *Biological Psychiatry Branch, National Institute of Mental Health, Bethesda, MD*

Richard H. Price • *University of Michigan, Institute for Social Research, Ann Arbor, MI*

Marc I. Rosen • *Connecticut Mental Health Center, New Haven, CT*

Jean B. Strohl • *RAPPORT, Inc., Chevy Chase, MD*

Lorand B. Szalay • *RAPPORT, Inc., Chevy Chase, MD*

Jalie A. Tucker • *Department of Psychology, Auburn University, Auburn, AL*

Shelley K. Vilov • *RAPPORT, Inc., Chevy Chase, MD*

Rudy E. Vuchinich • *Department of Psychology, Auburn University, Auburn, AL*
Barbara C. Wallace • *Department of Health Education, Teachers College, Columbia University, New York*
Susan R. B. Weiss • *Biological Psychiatry Branch, National Institute of Mental Health, Bethesda, MD*

Drug Abuse Treatment

M. Douglas Anglin and Yih-Ing Hser

Introduction

Illicit drug use has had profound economic and cultural effects on American society, contributing to sharp increases in the crime rate, accelerating the spread of AIDS, and diverting some minority groups from the economic mainstream. The primary response of government agencies has been increased effort to reduce crime rates by preventing the spread of drug use to uninitiated populations and interdicting the flow of drugs into the United States.[1–3] Such approaches have been both costly and limited in effect, however,[4] and alternatives, especially reducing demand for drugs by treating drug addicts, are increasingly promoted. A growing body of evidence indicates that demand reduction efforts directed toward those seriously involved represents a far more cost-effective method for reducing drug use, the user's criminal activities, and the resulting burden on society.[5–11]

However, demand reduction through the treatment of drug abuse is not without policy and practical limitations. A careful review of the research literature allows several definitive conclusions to be drawn. First, and most obvious, there is no simple cure for drug dependence. More than 50 years of studies have shown that, once drug dependence has developed, the problem persists as a chronic condition, and relapse is common. Biological, sociocultural, economic, and psychological factors have all been identified as contributors to drug abuse either individually or in

From: *Drug and Alcohol Abuse Reviews, Vol. 4: Drug Abuse Treatment*
Ed: R. R. Watson ©1992 The Humana Press Inc.

combination. The treatment of drug abuse is thus not a simple medical issue, but involves a wide spectrum of social considerations. The complications of treating drug abusers include alcohol abuse, polydrug use, psychiatric disorders, criminal involvement, and social dysfunction (e.g., unemployment and homelessness).

Treatment of heroin abuse has been most thoroughly documented because that has been the primary drug of abuse in the past and because of its clear link to criminal activity.[12–17] More recently, however, cocaine abuse has become one of the nation's major drug problems, receiving increasing public and research attention,[18] and its use has also been linked to the rising crime rate.[19–21] Although few studies of treatment efficacy have focused specifically on cocaine abusers, some researchers are concluding that fundamental similarities in the addiction processes for heroin and cocaine make results obtained with the former directly applicable to the latter.[22]

Four major treatment modalities are now used in the treatment of heroin addicts. *Detoxification* (detox) programs are concerned with the medical management of symptoms associated with drug withdrawal. If they are not used in combination with other treatment regimens, these programs provide only minimal long-term therapeutic benefits. Their most common use is for amelioration of drug craving as a "gateway" to other, more intensive treatment interventions. *Methadone maintenance* (MM) programs substitute a licit opiate under controlled conditions for illicit opiates, such as heroin. Despite controversy about the morality of such substitution, MM has become the dominant modality for the treatment of opiate addicts and has been most frequently evaluated. *Therapeutic community* (TC) programs provide a controlled residential environment with intensive personality restructuring efforts. TCs have been typically applied to heroin addicts, but are increasingly used for other drugs and comprise the second most frequently evaluated modality. Because of low controversy and low cost factors, *outpatient drug-free* (ODF) programs providing drug education and counseling have increased considerably in numbers, though evaluation studies of their effectiveness are essentially lacking. These four modalities accounted for more than 90% of all clients in treatment as of 1987.[23]

In recent years, many physicians have also begun using *28-d inpatient programs* for the treatment of cocaine abuse. Such programs were originally designed for the treatment of alcohol abuse, but by the mid-1980s, more than half the patients in such programs were cocaine abusers.[24] Their goal is to remove the addict from the environment that triggered dependence and, with intensive treatment, to allow clients to break through their defenses and confront their denial. Combinations of these predominant treatment regimens, the so-called mixed-modality programs, have shown promise in bettering outcomes, but such combinations have not been implemented except in isolated circumstances.[25]

The lack of determinant criteria has hindered the optimal matching of clients to treatment programs to ensure the greatest rates of success and cost–benefit return for a given treatment episode.[26] Neither has it been possible to identify factors that consistently predict posttreatment abstinence or relapse patterns. In general, treatment success is relatively independent of race, sex, ethnic origins, and socioeconomic status.[22] Evidence also indicates that individuals coerced into treatment benefit as much as those who enter treatment voluntarily,[22] but dropout rates are high for all modalities except some MM programs. A significant proportion of those seeking treatment do not stay in treatment, especially in TCs and ODF, for more than a few weeks. Clients entering all treatment modalities under legal coercion are thought to remain in treatment longer.

Typically, an intact marriage, a job, shorter drug use history, low levels of psychiatric dysfunctioning, and a history of minimal criminality predict a better outcome in most programs.[22] For some individuals, especially those with high levels of criminal involvement and high psychopathology, treatment is of limited benefit when applied for brief periods. Demographic characteristics, such as sex, race/ethnicity, or education, are related to the likelihood of entering treatment, but are of limited use in predicting treatment outcomes. Older age at treatment admission has been consistently found to be positively associated with better treatment outcome. Generally, relationships found between patient characteristics and outcome, although reliable across studies in their effects, often explain only a small amount of the outcome variations within treatment programs.

Treatment in the Community

The simplistic treatment goal has traditionally been to intervene so that the drug abuser stops using drugs. The ultimate behavioral objectives from society's point of view are manifold, however, driven by social concerns, such as crime reduction, prison management, and more recently, reducing the spread of AIDS.[27] Additional goals include improving the social and personal functioning of the client.

In examining the efficacy of treatment, therefore, it is important that studies employ outcome measures assessing multiple behavior domains, rather than focusing solely on whether clients stopped using drugs. The outcome of treatment, usually measured by discrete and incomplete variables, is actually a dynamic result of interrelated performances in several domains. The most important outcomes include:

1. Cessation or decreased use of the primary drug of dependence or other drugs;
2. Decreased level of illegal activities, such as drug trafficking, property crime, or prostitution;
3. Increased employment and decreased reliance on social service agencies;
4. Improved social and family functioning;
5. Improved psychological functioning; and
6. Decreased mortality and improved physical health.

Some researchers include the additional category of increased program retention.[28] Demonstrable improvements in these areas are valuable treatment achievements and should be considered as important measures of efficacy along with the issue of drug abstinence.

A variety of different behavioral factors have been associated with increased or reduced efficacy of drug abuse treatment. For example, using multidimensional assessments of multiple outcomes of 123 opiate addicts followed for 6 mo after admission, Rounsaville et al.[29] found that outcome is predicted with relative accuracy by initial functioning in the behavioral domain examined. For example, previous work history predicts employment during the follow-up period, history of imprisonments and antisocial personality predict illegal activity, pretreatment duration of opiate addiction predicts illicit drug use, and initial psychiatric symptom level and depressive diagnosis predict symptom status at follow-up. No single predictor was significantly related to all of the outcome factors. Other studies have also consistently shown that clients with more criminal involvement before treatment have the poorest outcomes.[30–32] Other negative prognoses include alcohol use[33–37] and polydrug use,[38,39] unemployment,[40,41] and dual diagnosis.[34,42–44] Among these factors, psychopathology has been studied most extensively and has been identified as influential in treatment outcome.

Research has been accumulated to show a high degree of psychopathology displayed by drug addicts. McLellan et al.[45,46] in Philadelphia demonstrated the importance of psychopathology in relation to treatment outcome. They reported that the severity of psychological problems at admission is a powerful predictor of several outcome criteria, such as illicit drug use, criminal activity, social productivity, and psychological adjustment, when these are measured 6 mo after entry into treatment.

Evaluations of major programs and modalities have typically been conducted either as individual programs or as part of large-scale, multimodality studies. Large-scale studies conducted in recent years include nationally oriented data bases, such as the Drug Abuse Reporting Program (DARP) and the Treatment Outcome Prospective Study (TOPS). DARP contains client information on 44,000 clients entering 52 treatment agencies from 1969 to 1973. Several major follow-up studies were conducted at 1, 3, 6, and 12 yr following DARP treatment. As a successor to DARP, TOPS included 11,750 clients who entered 41 drug abuse treatment programs in 10 cities nationwide during 1979–1981. Follow-up studies of subsamples of these cohorts have been undertaken, ranging from 3–60 mo after termination of treatment.[40] Common findings from the literature or treatment effectiveness are presented below for the predominant modalities.

Detoxification

This modality provides a short-term use of licit drugs (such as antidepressants, methadone, or buprenorphine) that focuses on withdrawal from illicit drugs and the medical management of symptoms. Other than referral to other treatment services, detox usually provides no subsequent therapeutic services. Most detox programs focus on narcotics dependence and use methadone to establish a staged withdrawal, typically over 21 d. Research findings are available only for opioid detoxification.

The primary objective of opioid detoxification treatment is to provide symptomatic relief from the opioid abstinence syndrome while physical dependence on opioids is being eliminated. Methadone is the only opioid drug currently approved for treating opiate dependence and is the detoxification agent routinely employed. The patient is first stabilized on a dose of methadone sufficient to prevent withdrawal symptoms and is then detoxified by stepwise reductions in the daily dose.

No data support the long-term efficacy of detox. This treatment, however, is effective in reducing drug use temporarily, and there is a demand for it. Senay[47] pointed out that, from a clinical point of view, detoxification programs are needed to treat emergent episodes, reduce the length and severity of "runs," and attract addicts into the treatment system.

Methadone Maintenance

In general, MM is intended for those patients who have already attempted drug-free forms of treatment, and for whom there is little or no expectation that they will be able to function normally without chemotherapeutic support.[48] Because methadone is itself addictive, clients can be maintained in the program as long as desired if program rules are followed and if funding is maintained. Some jurisdictions, however, have terminated methadone programs or provided funding for only limited-duration MM. In these areas, clients must pay the full cost of treatment.

Most MM programs are in outpatient settings. The structure used by most programs includes explicit rules for behavior (with treatment discharge often being a consequence of infractions), mandatory counseling sessions, routine urine testing, and medications taken under direct supervision. Structure and support services vary from program to program (e.g., amount of counseling services, dosage level, and retention policy).[49]

MM has been subjected to the most extensive evaluation of any modality. Positive outcomes have been obtained in most studies, including DARP, TOPS, and other individual program evaluations. Several reviews[12,13,50] provide broad evidence that MM consistently produces significant decreases in both opioid use and criminality, as well as improvements in general health. Even when addicts are discharged from treatment, some sustained improvement is still observable, although to a lesser degree when compared to effects while in treatment.[51] Anglin and his colleagues,[51,52] for example, have shown that the percentage of nonincarcerated time engaged in daily narcotics use decreased from about 70% (averaging across several studies) when not in MM treatment to about 12% when in an MM program. The percentage of time abstinent from narcotics increased from about 12% to about 26% and, likewise, the property crime involvement decreased from about 18% when not in MM to about 11% when in MM.

Other examples that highlight the effectiveness of MM treatment in reducing crime are available. Maddux and Desmond[54] studied the association between community crime rates and the rate of institutional and

MM treatment in the San Antonio area. They found that, as treatment rates increased, community crime rates decreased; when cutbacks forced the premature discharge of patients, community crime rates increased. Ball et al.[9] examined six MM programs located in New York City, Philadelphia, and Baltimore. MM was found to be effective for the 671 subjects studied in reducing illicit drug use and crime during treatment. The reduction in criminality was dramatic; the average 307 crime days/person/yr during the addiction period prior to treatment was reduced to 18–24 crime days/person/yr when in treatment after 6 mo. Similar findings have been reported by McLellan et al.[55] at the Philadelphia Veterans Administration Medical Center, by Burt et al.[56] in New York City and Washington DC, and by Anglin and McGlothlin[52] in Southern California, among many others.

These reported outcome results are impressive, but the lack of control groups in all of these studies makes a strict quantification of the positive results ambiguous. For example, some degree of improvement might have occurred as a result of the passage of time, age, and so on. Results from several "natural experiments" are available, however, and have generated a unique depiction of the effects of the termination of entire treatment programs.[57] Also apparent in the results from these studies are the overall costs and benefits of the substitution of fee-for-service methadone programs for those supported by public funds.[58] A study of the effects of involuntary termination of MM was possible when a Bakersfield, CA clinic was closed in 1976 by local officials.[59] A 2-yr follow-up study compared behavior between the 94 methadone clients forced to be discharged from the Bakersfield clinic with a matched sample of 83 clients obtained from the Tulare, CA clinic, where no such policy was enforced. The results showed that 54% of the terminated clients became readdicted to heroin, and the arrest and incarceration rates were approximately double those for the comparison sample.

A similar policy change occurred in San Diego, CA in 1978, although, unlike the Bakersfield clinic closure where no alternative programs were established, San Diego allowed private MM providers to open clinics. For those who transferred to private MM after the closure of a clinic, fewer differences were observed. Major adverse consequences were found for clients unable or unwilling to transfer to private programs: Higher crime and dealing rates, more contact with the criminal justice system, and higher rates of illicit drug use were demonstrated by nontransfer clients.[58]

Even with the majority of the results demonstrating positive treatment outcome, MM has been and still is a controversial approach to treating heroin addiction. Major issues include detoxification from methadone as a treatment goal, dosage effects, take-home policies, street diversion, and so forth. Several studies suggest that adequate dosage levels of methadone are necessary to ensure retention in the program and to achieve desired results. McGlothlin and Anglin[59] and Fisher and Anglin,[60] for example, compared three MM programs, two of which used high doses (i.e., a mean stabilization dose of 82–95 mg), whereas the third used low doses (i.e., a mean of 43 mg) and a relatively strict policy with respect to involuntary termination for program violations. The study showed that, for the two high-dose programs, retention was much longer than for the low-dose program (at 2 yr after treatment entry, approx 40 and 70% of clients remained in the two high-dose programs, whereas only 20% remained in the low-dose program). During the 6–7-yr period from program entry to interview, the clients from the two high-dose programs also had significantly fewer arrests and less incarceration, narcotic addiction, and self-reported criminal behavior than did the clients in the low-dose program. These benefits persisted until the time of interview, and were present whether the client was on or off methadone.

Little work on the effects of take-home policy has been reported. Stitzer[61] studied the use of take-home privileges as a reinforcement for attendance at counseling sessions. She found that attendance increased significantly above the levels observed during the period of noncontingency. Milby et al.[62] and Stitzer et al.[63] concluded that methadone take-home privileges can be powerful reinforcers of rehabilitative behaviors.

Therapeutic Community

TC treatment is conducted in a residential facility; treatment involves personality restructuring within a highly structured environment and focuses on social relationship development. Examples of this type of approach include the early Synanon model and subsequent programs, such as Daytop Village,[64] Phoenix House, and Gateway House.[65] The treatment does not include any chemical agent, except for medical or psychiatric reasons. The primary treatment approach includes encounter-group therapy, tutorial learning sessions, remedial and formal education classes, residential job duties, and in later stages, conventional occupations for live-in/work-out clients.[66] This therapy involves a highly demanding, 24-hours-a-day social setting, with patient-government and group pressures to socialize the individual into accepting more adaptive attitudes as well as patterns of productive behavior. The optimal residential stay varies across programs, but traditional TCs require at least 15 mo in residence for completion. Some TCs, however, have incorporated shorter periods of stay (e.g., 6–12 mo) based on clients' needs and progress.[66] Success is defined as a change to a lifestyle that is drug-free, economically productive, and free from antisocial behavior.

Both DARP and TOPS, as well as other reviews of evaluation research in TCs, found that the modality produced significant improvement in immediate and long-term outcome status of the clients.[67] Drug use and criminality declined, whereas measures of prosocial behavior (employment and/or school involvement) increased.[68–79]

Program evaluation studies of TC clients are best represented by De Leon's research on the Phoenix House.[80–82] The Phoenix House Program in New York City is the nation's largest TC drug-free treatment system. The program treats all types of substance abuse, although the majority (80%) of clients are heroin addicts. Evaluation studies of immediate and long-term outcome status of the clients treated showed significant improvement compared to pretreatment status. Drug use and criminality declined, whereas measures of prosocial behavior (employment and/or school involvement) increased.[67] Studies examining differences between clients who completed treatment (graduated) and those who dropped out indicated that the graduates were significantly better than dropouts in all measures of outcome.

Studies analyzing the time in the program for TC dropouts report a positive relationship between favorable outcome and length of stay in treatment.[67,69,71–73,78,79] The magnitude of the changes varied across studies, and several studies with positive outcome findings failed to obtain time-in-program differences.[70] The likelihood of retention is difficult to predict from client characteristics, however.

Outpatient Drug-Free Treatment

This type of program includes a wide variety of outpatient nonmaintenance programs. In the early 1970s, ODF was mainly for youthful nonopiate users. Subsequently, almost as many opiate addicts have entered ODF as MM programs. Whether programs are oriented toward the treatment of opiates or nonopiates, the same services are typically provided in both types. Treatment regimens usually do not rely on any chemical agent or medication, but prescription drugs can be used as an adjunct to treatment or to treat medical problems. Temporary use of drugs (e.g., use of tranquilizers for psychiatric disorders) is permissible. The primary treatment approach employs outpatient services relying on counseling and training in social skills. ODF programs vary widely, ranging from highly demanding daytime TCs to relaxed programs of recreational activities. The planned duration usually is short-term, and referral is made to community agencies for health, mental health, education, vocational, legal, housing, financial, family, and other required services. This treatment emphasizes abstinence from both licit and illicit drugs with attention paid to life circumstances that foster drug use.

Evaluations based on DARP data generally indicate that ODF is less effective than MM or TC in retaining clients, but is just as effective in other, long-term behavioral outcomes. The number of patients that ODF serves, however, was usually small. Furthermore, the favorable results for ODF were restricted to "nonaddicts," clients who used opioids less than daily, usually in conjunction with other drugs, or who used only nonopioids.

Results based on TOPS data show that ODF clients were most likely to leave treatment in the first 1 (21%) to 4 wk (36%).[30] By 3 mo after treatment entry, more than 60% had dropped out, transferred, or completed treatment. Among the three major modalities that TOPS examined, ODF clients were also the least successful in reducing their drug use. About a third of those classified as more than minimal users at admission had continued or increased use after 3 mo in treatment, although 45% of users reported a large reduction in use. ODF was also less successful at reducing crime among clients; about one in four clients who had reported an illegal act before treatment continued involvement in illegal activities.

28-d Inpatient Programs

Although there have been no well controlled evaluations of the 28-d programs, some follow-up information exists for one sample of cocaine abusers. Rawson et al.[83] conducted 1-yr follow-up interviews with a group of 65 cocaine abusers treated at the Sierra Tucson center in Arizona. The population consisted primarily of single, male, Anglo cocaine abusers with relatively short drug histories. During the first year after discharge from Sierra Tucson, 32% of the cocaine abusers returned to monthly or more frequent cocaine use. An additional 23% returned to regular use of alcohol or other drugs. Overall, 45% of the cocaine abusers treated in the program gave self-reports of achieving 1 yr of abstinence successfully, compared to 75% of alcoholics graduating from the program.

One clear conclusion of the study was that return to alcohol use was a strong predictor for cocaine relapse. Among the cocaine users who resumed drinking after graduation from the program, cocaine use occurred in 61%.[83] Among those who had refrained from alcohol use, only 8% relapsed to cocaine use. Currently, several different studies are evaluating the efficacy of 28-d programs.

Comparisons Among Treatment Modalities

Although the general effectiveness of treatment is widely supported and accepted, less conclusive findings are available addressing the differential effectiveness among the existing treatment modalities. Clients' self-selection into different programs makes direct outcome comparisons among treatments difficult, and research results often need careful qualification. Some studies have, however, used an experimental design that attempted to resolve this issue, though with limited success.

A representative treatment evaluation comparison between MM and three TCs using an experimental design was reported by Bale et al.[84] They studied 585 heroin-addicted male veterans who were randomly assigned to either MM or one of three TCs after a 5-d detoxification program. Subjects were followed up at 6 mo and at 1 yr. Data were collected on drug use, criminal behavior, and work and school attendance. Only 108 of the subjects accepted the random assignment and spent as long as 1 wk in their assigned program, however. Most subjects dropped out early in treatment, especially from the TC programs. Less than 50% of clients remained in the programs 2 mo after admission.

There were no outcome differences between the combined results from the three TC groups and those from the MM group, however, at either follow-up period. Because of the high dropout rate, the outcome differences between the two modalities were virtually uninterpretable. The subjects who remained in a TC longer than 50 d, however, did consistently better than the MM group at 1-yr follow-up.

The multimodality nature of DARP and TOPS allows some limited comparison among modalities. DARP contrasted treatment outcomes for MM, TC, ODF, and detoxification against an intake-only (IO) group of subjects who were eligible for and admitted to a waiting list, but who did not subsequently enter treatment as scheduled. The DARP studies showed that actual retention in treatment for all DARP clients was shorter overall than most clients had anticipated at entry. The median time in treatment was over 12 mo in MM, between 3 and 4 mo in TC and ODF, and <2 wk in detoxification.[31]

At follow-up, behavioral changes related to drug use, criminal involvement, and employment in the first 1–3 yr after treatment were consistently better for clients in MM, TC, and ODF programs than for those in the detoxification and IO groups. The outcome differences among the three effective treatments were not significant, however. For example, in the first year post-DARP, 27% of the MM, 28% of the TC, and 24% of the ODF clients used no illicit drugs and had no arrests or time in prison, as compared to 15% of the detoxification and 14% of the IO clients.[85] In agreement with other research, the DARP studies also found that clients who remained in treatment longer and who demonstrated more favorable performance during treatment tended to have more favorable posttreatment outcomes. There also appeared to be a minimum time in treatment for any favorable results: Clients in MM, TC, and ODF who remained <3 mo had relatively poor outcomes comparable with those in the detoxification group, regardless of the reason for termination. Differences for the opiate addict samples among all modalities diminished over the 12-yr follow-up, understandably, because other subsequent intervening influences would have been operational.[86]

Treatment evaluation results from TOPS contrasted the same four modalities, and generally supported those from DARP and other studies. Detoxification clients showed the least effective outcomes overall, and the short duration in treatment precluded more refined analysis. Dropout rates were high across all drug treatment modalities.[30] By 3 mo in treatment, <40% of ODF clients remained in treatment (36% dropped out during the first month). The comparable numbers were 65% for MM and 44% for TC clients. Outcomes during the first 3 mo in treatment showed that >95% of retained TC clients and 80% of MM clients reported reduced use of their primary drug. ODF clients were the least successful in reducing their drug use; only about 45% reported a large reduction in use.

Illegal predatory activity was common in the pretreatment period among all clients in the TOPS study, but was most frequent among TC clients. During the first 3 mo in treatment, about 70% of the retained MM and ODF clients who had predatory activity before treatment reported cessation of this behavior during treatment. The reports of TC clients plummeted. Of TC clients who had pretreatment involvement in such activity, 97% reported cessation during treatment.

The posttreatment outcomes measured in the year after terminating treatment showed major improvement in drug use and criminal activities for the three major modalities, although the improvement was smaller than that which occurred during the treatment program. Those clients who remained in treatment longer (at least 3 mo) appeared to have more positive outcomes. The greatest posttreatment reduction in illegal predatory activity occurred for TC clients. Although 60% reported at least one predatory act in the year before TOPS treatment, only one-third reported such activity in the year after treatment. Smaller decreases in illegal activity were reported for MM and ODF clients. About 5–10% of the clients in all modalities continued to commit a high number of predatory crimes after discharge.

Treatment in the Criminal Justice System

Drug use is extensive among individuals who come into contact with the criminal justice system (CJS). Results from the nationwide Drug Use Forecasting study[86] conducted in a number of major cities have shown, for example, that urine tests of arrestees indicate high rates of illicit drug use. Illicit drugs were detected in the urine of 40–70% of arrestees, depending on the city. As would be expected, these high rates are echoed in probation and correctional samples. Studies of prison inmates indicate that from 40–80% report serious substance abuse histories.[87,88]

As a consequence of the high numbers of drug abusing offenders involved with the CJS, many programs of diversion, corrections-based drug education and treatment, and probation and parole supervision programs designed for the drug abuser have been developed. Typically, such programs are short-lived—developed under one administration and terminated under subsequent ones. The most recent full cycle of interest in such programs developed in the early 1970s, but of those established, most had terminated by the late 1970s.[88,89] A new cycle of interest and program development was initiated in the late 1980s, and is likely to continue throughout the 1990s.

Some authors have believed that little benefit can be derived when a client is forced into treatment by the CJS.[90–92] Other authors have argued that few chronic addicts would enter treatment without such external motivation and that legal coercion is as justified as any other motivation for treatment entry. Moreover, some empirical evidence suggests that the CJS consequences that can result from failure to meet treatment program conditions may lead to more socially acceptable behavior than is produced by treatment alone.[93–96] Those who contend that a purely voluntary treatment system would not attract a significant number of addicts also argue that controlling addiction benefits society as a whole; that is, the judicial system *should* bring addicts into treatment to safeguard the interests and well-being of the community.[38,41,97]

Civil Commitment

Several different approaches to linking drug treatment and criminal justice interventions have been attempted during the last 70 years. One of the earliest efforts was civil commitment, which proved to be an extremely strong approach. Civil commitment is a legal procedure that allows the commitment of narcotics addicts or other drug addicts to a compulsory drug treatment program, typically, but not necessarily, involving a residential period and a community-based aftercare period. Provisions are often included for helping clients with education and employment needs, and for responding promptly to signs of readdiction—usually detected by regular urinalysis monitoring. Civil commitment is frequently used with addicts who are arrested for criminal activity. With criminal charges pending, the addict can be coerced into treatment and retained long enough to receive the benefits of a treatment program.

This approach is particularly attractive because it provides the benefits of rehabilitation for the addict while simultaneously reducing demand for drugs during both the treatment and the aftercare phases. Both outcomes result in the socially desirable goal of reducing the drug dealing activities and property crimes that support illicit drug habits.

Several studies of the California Civil Addict Program (CAP) illustrate the effectiveness of in-prison and follow-up treatment. The first study compared heroin addicts who were admitted to the program and subsequently released into the community under supervision for up to 7 yr with addicts who were discharged from the program after a short period because of legal errors in the commitment procedures.[98] During the 7 yr after commitment, the program group reduced daily narcotics use by 21.8%, whereas the discharged group reduced daily use by only 6.8%.

Furthermore, criminal activities among the commitment group were reduced by 18.6%, whereas the discharged group reported a reduction of only 6.7%.

A second evaluation[99] identified three subsamples of CAP admissions according to narcotics use and treatment status at the time of the interview, some 12 yr after admission to the program: a "maturing out" sample,[100] a "subsequent treatment" sample, and a "chronic street addict" sample. The maturing out sample, about 40% of the total, had steadily reduced daily narcotic consumption during the commitment period and did not resume addicted use after discharge. At the time of the interview, many subjects in this sample occasionally used narcotics, but few were addicted.

The subsequent treatment sample, about 30% of the total, showed a large decrease (approx 20–25%) in daily narcotics use during the commitment period. After discharge, however, addicted use rapidly increased. Three years after discharge, addicted use by this group had reached precommitment levels. Addicted use continued at that resumed level until the group reentered long-term treatment, this time with MM. Daily use decreased dramatically for this group after admission to MM.

The chronic street addict sample, approx 30% of the program group, showed a moderate reduction (7–10%) in daily narcotic use during the commitment period. After discharge, addicted use levels rose to a level exceeding that reported in the precommitment period and was still high in the year preceding the interview; for that year, the chronic street addicts described themselves as being addicted 55% of their nonincarcerated time, as compared to approx 4% of the maturing out sample and 8% of the MM sample.

These studies have two important findings. First, civil commitment as implemented in the California CAP reduced daily narcotic use and associated property crime by program participants to one-third the levels displayed by similar addicts who were not in the program. Second, although the program's effects differed across three types of addicts, narcotics use and crime were suppressed in all three groups. Therefore, a conclusion is warranted that the program was generally effective in reducing demand for heroin.

Unfortunately, these results were not available to California corrections planners in a timely fashion. During the 1970s, budgetary pressures led not only to a cutback in the number of convicts enrolled in the program, but also to cutbacks in or the removal of some of the most effective elements of the program, including training of personnel, the time spent in the program, and monitoring of clients. Thus, although it was still utilized, the CAP became little more than a shell of the former program, and its value as a corrective tool declined correspondingly.

Similar positive results have been obtained in other studies of CJS-based drug treatment efforts. In a study of a therapeutic community in a New York state prison, for example, Wexler et al.[101] found that only 27% of the subjects in the therapeutic community were rearrested while on parole, compared to about 40% of those not treated. Furthermore, for those who were arrested, the time until arrest was significantly longer for those treated in the therapeutic community. Finally, a meta-analysis of 80 different studies[102] showed that appropriately designed and implemented drug abuse interventions in prisons produced a significantly lower rate of recidivism than did no treatment or poorly applied treatment. Treatment was found to be effective in both adults and juveniles, in studies before and after 1980, in randomized and nonrandomized designs, and in diversionary, community, and residential programs.

The TASC Program

Some states have developed coordinated programs to refer drug abusing offenders to community-based treatment programs in lieu of prosecution or probation revocation. One such program, called Treatment Alternatives to Street Crime (TASC), was initiated in 1972 and grew to include programs in a majority of states. By 1988, however, programs were in operation in only 18 states.[103] Under TASC auspices, community-based treatment is made available for drug-dependent individuals who otherwise might become progressively more involved with the CJS. To motivate drug offenders to enter and remain in treatment, TASC employs diversionary dispositions, such as deferred prosecution, creative community sentencing, and pretrial intervention. Dropping out of treatment or other noncompliance is treated by the courts as a violation of the conditions of release.

Evaluations of the impact of TASC have been limited.[97] Most TASC programs, however, are believed to have performed the treatment-outreach function successfully. Sells[104] for example, reports that 50% of the referrals entered treatment for the first time. Some independent local evaluations have also concluded that local TASC programs effectively intervened with clients to reduce drug abuse and criminal activity.[104]

The most extensive—albeit still limited—evaluations of the impact of TASC or similar programs are based on the TOPS study.[38,105] These studies compared CJS-involved clients (in TASC and under other forms of justice-system supervision) to voluntary drug treatment clients in terms of demographic characteristics, treatment retention, treatment progress, and predatory behavior in the year following treatment termination. TASC clients improved as much as voluntary clients with respect to drug use, employment, and criminal behavior during the first 6 mo of treatment. TASC clients also tended to remain in both residential and outpatient drug-free modalities 6–7 wk longer than did voluntary clients or those under other CJS referrals—a finding usually associated with better treatment outcomes.[97] The monitoring functions of TASC seem to have encouraged this longer treatment participation.

Evaluations of CJS-Mandated Treatment

Studies have shown that legal pressure increases admission rates into treatment programs and may promote better retention in treatment, consequently improving the overall results of the program. McFarlain et al.,[106] for example, found that legal pressure increased retention during the first 30 d after admission, but not long-term retention. Similarly, Schnoll et al.[107] found that legal pressure increased retention in an inpatient treatment program and that clients admitted immediately after release from prison were most likely to complete the program.

Longitudinal data from DARP indicate that coercion does not impair the effectiveness of treatment programs. Sells and associates[108–110] and Simpson and Friend[111] examined the relationship between contact with the CJS at admission and length of stay in treatment, as well as client performance during and after treatment. These studies found that those entering treatment with some legal involvement performed as well as those who entered voluntarily. The studies also showed, unlike the TOPS findings, that legal status was not a significant contributor to retention, as indicated by discriminate functions estimated separately for MM, ODF programs, and short-term TC programs.

Similarly, Anglin et al.[112] compared three groups of heroin addicts, totaling 296 individuals, who entered MM under high, moderate, or low coercion levels. They found no significant difference among the groups in the improvement levels of drug use and criminal behavior. These groups could not be distinguished in terms of their behaviors, indicating that those coerced into treatment benefited just as much as those entering voluntarily.

More recently, Anglin and Powers[113] studied 202 MM clients who had experienced each of four different treatment regimens during their addiction careers: MM alone, legal supervision (probation or parole) with drug testing alone, both interventions simultaneously, and neither intervention. Legal supervision with drug testing was found to be better than no intervention in improving the drug-related behavior of narcotics addicts, and MM alone was markedly better than legal supervision. The combination of MM and legal supervision was at least as good as MM alone, and was better with regard to abstinence from narcotics use. The study also showed no differences in effectiveness of the therapies with respect to gender or ethnicity, suggesting that the combination of legal supervision and MM should be effective for any group.

Benefit/Cost Analysis

Remarkably few researchers have attempted to perform benefit/cost analyses for drug abuse treatment, perhaps because the benefits are exceptionally hard to quantify. The detailed categories of the consequences of drug abuse that may be attenuated by treatment include: reduced medical expenditures on drug-related illness; increased school or labor productivity; reduced amounts of property stolen by drug abusers to support their habits; reduced private costs of crime-prevention measures to deter and detect such thefts (e.g., alarms, locks, security devices, and so on); reduced anxiety and fears stemming from the possibility of victimization; reduced levels of abuse and other emotional and physical harm imposed on the children, parents, and spouses of drug abusers; reduced public expenditures for police, courts, and corrections to detect and process drug violations and property crimes committed by drug abusers; reduced public expenditures to treat drug-related illnesses, including overdoses, hepatitis, and AIDS; reduced welfare payments made to drug users and their families; and reduced loss of tax revenues because of lower productivity and reduced labor-market participation by drug users.

The reduction in these consequences constitutes a large measure of the benefits of drug abuse treatment and other intervention programs, and provides the rationale for their support by public funds. Harwood et al.,[114] for example, estimated the economic impact on society of drug abuse in 1983 to be close to $57 billion. A substantial part of the total was attributed to reduced productivity and crime. A later study reported that the annual national expenditure on illicit drugs had risen far above \$60 billion in 1989.[115] Increased medical expenses for crack addicts and their infants and drug-related AIDS cases seem to be causing a significant portion of the rising expense.

Surprisingly little is known about the actual costs of delivering drug abuse treatment.[116] Some crude estimates of direct costs, without amortization, suggest that, per person, the cost of residential treatment is about three times the cost of outpatient MM or ODF treatment.[40,116]

Several techniques are available for combining estimates of costs and benefits.[117] A commonly used method is to form a benefit/cost ratio to quantify efficacy. If, for example, 1 yr of treatment for a heroin addict in a therapeutic community costs \$8000 and this results in \$24,000 in benefits to society, then the benefit/cost ratio is 3. A ratio in excess of 1 would indicate efficiency at a level necessary to rationalize continuation of a program—although other factors may come into consideration as well.

One analysis that examined economic benefits to society utilized data from the 1980 TOPS.[40,114] This analysis focused on the economic benefits derived from a decrease in criminal activity during treatment and 1 yr after discharge. The benefit/cost ratio of treatment was compared across three treatment modalities based on average length of stay and was found to be higher than 1 for both TC and ODF programs. Wallack[116] also found that the aggregate costs of treatment amount to <3% of the total cost of drug abuse to society.

Anglin et al.[58] investigated the effects of involuntary termination of MM when a San Diego clinic was closed. Some of the clients were able to transfer to privately funded programs, whereas others were unable or unwilling to do so. Those who were unable to transfer into private MM programs had higher crime and drug-dealing rates, more contact with the CJS, and higher rates of illicit drug use. The mean annual societal costs for male clients transferred into other programs was \$4031 compared to \$10,982 for those who were not transferred. Comparable figures for women were \$3881 and \$9689. The savings resulting from closing the MM program were thus offset by increased costs for incarceration, legal supervision, and other government-funded drug treatment.

McGlothlin and Anglin,[59] as discussed earlier, compared three MM programs. Two programs, A and B, used relatively high doses of methadone, and had flexible program policies with respect to client management, discharge for program infractions, and degrees of supportive counseling.

Program C used low doses of methadone and had a relatively strict policy with respect to involuntary termination for program violations.

Retention was much longer in programs A and B than in program C. During the 6–7-yr period from program entry to interview, the clients from the former two programs had significantly fewer arrests and less incarceration, narcotic addiction, and self-reported criminal behavior than the clients in the low-dose program. These benefits persisted until the time of interview, and were present whether the client was on methadone or off. The social cost analysis among these programs calculated arrest, trial, incarceration, legal supervision, property crime losses, and welfare costs per year for the years from first daily narcotics use to program admission; then these same costs plus treatment costs were calculated per year for the years from treatment to follow-up. The estimated annual costs of subjects in these programs, as a percentage of pretreatment costs, were 47, 62, and 85%, respectively. Program A, the most expensive because of its long retention time, was also the most cost-effective, netting a 53% saving in social cost compared with only a 15% saving for program C.

This analysis deals only with the costs associated with the patients who were treated, raising the question of whether a program should have a shorter retention time so that more patients could be treated in each available slot, perhaps thereby making it more efficient. Hargreaves[118] took this slot fraction factor into account and extended the above social cost estimates to derive benefit/cost ratios for the three programs. The high-dose, long-retention programs still showed superior benefit/cost ratios (6.1, 4.5, and 2.7, for programs A, B, and C, respectively).

Elements of an Effective Program

Several program components and characteristics have been shown to be effective when appropriately implemented; notable components include psychotherapy, urine testing, legal coercion, and efforts to increase retention. A recent study[119] of 590 MM clients from the TOPS evaluation confirmed that a higher methadone dosage level, more frequent urine testing, and more frequent dosage take-home privileges were correlated with longer treatment retention and lower relapse rates. Other important program characteristics are treatment philosophy, program policies, qualifications of staff, and other quality-of-care aspects. Research into the effects of program components and characteristics have been sparse.

Since 1970, most studies of *psychotherapy* for addicts have been performed with MM patients. In eight studies reviewed by O'Brian et al.,[120] opiate-dependent patients were randomly assigned to psychotherapy or to a treatment control condition, usually drug counseling. Six of the studies (75%) showed a better outcome for clients in psychotherapy than for those in the control group.

A similar study in New Haven, however, did not find a significant effect for psychotherapy.[121] The study evaluated short-term interpersonal psychotherapy—a brief psychodynamic therapy—for 72 MM clients diagnosed as having concurrent psychiatric disorders, such as anxiety or depression. The multiple-outcome measures included treatment attrition, number of urine positives for illegal drugs, number of arrests, psychiatric symptomology, personal and social functioning, and attainment of individual goals. Attrition was high in both the treated and control groups, and the evaluation showed few differences between the two groups.

The contrast between outcomes of the two studies suggests that the recruiting and implementation strategies of Woody et al.[122] should be considered in designing additional treatment trials. These strategies include integration of a broad range of services for clients early in treatment, and the integration of drug treatment and psychotherapy staff.

Monitoring of illicit drug use by *urine testing* has been a common practice in most drug treatment programs and in the CJS-supervised programs for known drug-using offenders.[123] Considerable evidence points to its effectiveness when linked to sanctions applied to those who test positive.[98] McGlothlin et al.[98] found that urine testing in CJS settings rather than in community-treatment settings, and in combination with intensive legal or other supervision with sanctions for detected drug use, was more effective than supervision without testing in reducing daily narcotics use and criminal activity by the narcotics users admitted to the California CAP. Similar results were obtained in later work with MM clients.[124,125] The most recent study showed that the combination of legal supervision and urine testing significantly suppressed both narcotics use and concurrent property crime, although the latter responded less dramatically.

Retention in a treatment program and the type of discharge are program characteristics that have been consistently related to client status at follow-up. These characteristics are valuable measures of a program's ability to maintain client contact and enhance prospects for a therapeutic relationship that facilitates positive treatment outcomes. With few exceptions, most studies on the length of treatment find that longer treatment retention is associated with reduced drug use and crime, and increased employment.[126–128] Simpson's[127,128] study of DARP data also suggests that a minimum duration in treatment is necessary for effective treatment. Treatments lasting <90 d appear to be of limited benefit, regardless of the type of treatment involved. Beyond 90 d, however, treatment outcome improves in direct relationship to the length of time spent in treatment.[97] These findings are consistent with results from studies of TC programs in the community by De Leon et al.,[71,129] TC programs in correctional settings,[101] and MM programs.[9]

Interpretations of these results are complicated, however, by the selective termination of patients with poorer prognoses.[130] Baekland and Lundwall,[131] for example, in their critical review of the literature, concluded that "remainers" are likely to be a more stable group initially, and this may make better treatment outcomes more probable. They had higher rates of pretreatment employment and fewer total arrests, and were slightly older than the dropouts. Furthermore, follow-up studies often show some degree of improvement in minimal treatment or untreated groups as a function of the passage of time.[56]

Since programs can exert influence only when patients are enrolled, retention has been viewed as an important goal of all treatments. Determinants of retention in treatment have not been thoroughly studied. There is, however, some evidence to suggest that those who exhibit greater psychological disturbance, particularly depression, are more likely to leave treatment prematurely.[46,132–134]

Several demographic variables have been found to be predictors of retention. In general, clients who are black, unmarried, polydrug abusers, unemployed, or who have longer conviction records appear more likely to drop out of treatment.[133] Sansone[135] found lower retention rates for women, Hispanics, and other nonblack minorities, and suggested that treatment programs be modified to serve the needs of those low-retention subgroups more effectively. De Leon,[136] however, claimed that correlates between clients' demographic characteristics and retention have been weak, whereas motivation, perception, and the client's readiness appear more relevant to retention. Sansone also found slightly higher retention for clients on readmission, regardless of age, sex, or racial background. Collins and Allison[105] reported that drug abusers who are legally coerced into treatment stay longer. McFarlain et al.[106] found that retention was positively related to legal pressure, but only in the initial phases of treatment. They also reported finding no relationship between retention and either age or race.

Other research suggests that a broad definition of retention may be needed. Simpson et al.[31] reported that 39% of MM clients and about one-fourth of the ODF clients returned to treatment within a year. This raises the question of whether, for many drug abusers, repeated exposure to treatment is more effective than one episode.[5] In this respect, the total time in treatment may be more important, when accrued across treatment episodes, than retention in a single program.

Program policies and staff characteristics of providers of treatment services are more diverse than the program modalities and components that are applied by those providers. Of all the aspects of treatment structure, program policy and its execution by staff are perhaps the least quantifiable (and least studied) in terms of their effects on treatment outcomes.[137] Nevertheless, clinical impressions by many observers concur that disparate outcomes are often a function of providers' policies and staffs' methods of implementing those policies. Different outcomes are noted even when comparing programs that are virtually identical in their components and structures.[138]

Limited evaluation data describe the influence of program policies and staff implementation. In one of the best examples, a study of three MM programs in Southern California[59,60] showed that positive results and retention in the program were directly related to the methadone dosage policy. Outcomes within TC programs also vary considerably. De Leon[65] reported 3-mo and 6-mo retention rates for seven TC programs in which the highest rates were 46 and 35%, and the lowest were 23 and 18%. Reasons reported by those leaving treatment prematurely included program factors, such as conflicts with staff and differing views of treatment. De Leon concluded that improved outcomes were influenced by relations between the overall treatment environment and specific treatment elements. He noted, however, that the effects on outcomes of variations in character of therapeutic communities have been only indirectly inferred, and he proposes that more program-based research be undertaken to make explicit the relationships between treatment environments and outcomes.

The connection between staff characteristics and treatment efficacy was also noted by Joe et al.[119] Positive outcomes were associated with higher professional quality of the staff involved in diagnosing clients at admission and in designing treatment plans.

Similar findings were also obtained by Ball[138] in his study of six MM programs in three East Coast cities. Wide variations in outcome were observed in programs of similar design. Results were partially attributable to intangible factors of program "personality" that were affected by staff attitudes and approaches. Ball's study included confidential interviews with program personnel, from which emerged a relationship between program "morale" and treatment effectiveness. The dynamic relationships among staff, clients, and program structures must be more completely examined in order to make the evaluation of this aspect of treatment more meaningful.

Conclusions and Social Policy Implications

The accumulated research on treatment for drug abuse, as reviewed in this chapter and summarized in other studies (particularly two NIDA monographs[12,13]), demonstrates significant declines in drug use and criminal behavior by drug-dependent clients as a result of treatment. Research findings have not yet provided adequate data to enable optimum assignment of specifically designed treatment protocols to individual clients. Evaluation studies do, however, provide substantial evidence of overall treatment efficacy, thereby creating a context for further research to address the issue of differential matching as a key aspect of any broadened treatment approach.

Four program features are of greatest importance in designing and implementing treatment efforts. First, the period of intervention must be a lengthy one, since drug dependence (especially in regard to heroin and cocaine) is typically a chronically relapsing condition. Except in a minority of cases, several rounds of treatment (possibly including episodes in several different modalities), aftercare, and relapse may be expected, and it is not unreasonable to assume that years of structured intervention will be necessary to control, reduce, or eliminate drug dependence in any given individual.

Second, programs must initially provide a significant level of structure—such as a residential stay in a controlled setting or very close monitoring in an outpatient setting—so that the user can be detoxified from illicit drugs and thoroughly assessed, after which an individual program plan can be instituted.

The initial period of close control should be followed by a carefully structured program of further treatment and subsequent aftercare. Objective monitoring for drug use (e.g., urine testing) may enhance outcomes by diminishing the likelihood of relapse, as demonstrated by treatment outcome studies for CJS populations where programs may lack many rehabilitative services. Even in programs with strong supportive services, where such monitoring may not obtain direct effects, drug testing results provide clinically useful information for treatment staff.[119] Other ancillary interventions—such as psychiatric care, psychological services, or job training—that encourage retention in treatment and in community aftercare and that prevent relapse should be effected on an individual basis.

The third aspect of an effective program is flexibility—no absolute mandates should determine client management. Some level of continued or substitute drug use may be expected from the majority of those in community programs, whether under CJS auspices or not.[98,99] Intermittent drug use that does not seriously disrupt the individual's program plan should be dealt with on an individual basis in the context of the addict's overall adjustment. Any detected readdiction, however, requires immediate program reaction, such as, in the case of heroin use, placement either in a residential setting for detoxification or in a treatment program employing methadone or naltrexone.

Finally, any intervention program must undergo regular evaluation to determine its level of effectiveness and to determine whether changing characteristics of clients require compensatory changes in the program. Program staff and policies must be kept current with developments in the treatment of drug dependence, so that suitable new methods can be adopted and staff adequately trained in their utilization.

Empirical assessments of the need for treatment in drug-dependent groups suggest a necessary increase in treatment services and options, as well as in legally coerced treatment for drug-using offenders. Because of the present climate of restricted treatment availability and regional variation in determining client eligibility, identified populations may not adequately represent the full range of drug-dependent individuals. Furthermore, program waiting lists and required client fees may discourage some users with dependence problems from entering treatment. The cumulative effect of such "selective filtering" processes can result in inflated estimates of treatment outcomes in some cases—nevertheless, treatment strategies must strive to accommodate a wider range of the drug-dependent population. An expanded treatment capacity will accrue aggregate benefits to society, and allow clients who desire to be or should be in treatment to benefit more readily from such services. Empirical findings also suggest that a complementary system of ancillary rehabilitation services will offer additional remediation of the consequences of drug abuse.

Adjuncts of treatment that enhance outcomes include a psychiatric evaluation and provision of appropriate psychotherapy; attention to polydrug use problems (perhaps through urine monitoring[139] to assure early detection and thus early intervention); and increased ancillary services.[9,140] The provision of sufficient alternative economic opportunities is important so that clients in treatment do not need to remain enmeshed in the drug abuse subculture of drug dealing, property crime, or other activities in order to provide for their economic needs. This aspect is particularly important for demonstrably disadvantaged groups, such as minorities and women—particularly women with responsibility for child-rearing. Finally, for CJS-identified drug users, imposed legal sanctions coupled with treatment services should be applied to control drug use and crime effectively among this population.

Acknowledgments

M. Douglas Anglin is Adjunct Associate Professor and Yih-Ing Hser is Adjunct Assistant Professor at the Neuropsychiatric Institute, University of California, Los Angeles. Partial support for this chapter was provided by Grant No. DA05544 from the National Institute on Drug Abuse and Grant No. 91-IJ-CX-K009 from the National Institute of Justice. Drs. Anglin and Hser are also supported by Research Scientist Development Awards (DA00146, DA00139, respectively) from the National Institute on Drug Abuse. Special thanks are owed to Tom Maugh for editorial assistance.

References

[1]M. G. Graham (1987) Controlling drug abuse and crime: A research update, *(NIJ Reports/SNI* 202). National Institute of Justice, US Dept. Of Justice, NIJ, Washington, DC.

[2]R. C. Newman (1983) Diversion of addicts from the criminal justice system

in treatment. Paper presented at the National Conference of Standards, Ethics, and Practice, November 5, New York.

[3]J. H. Jaffe (1979) The swinging pendulum: The treatment of drug users in America, in *Handbook on Drug Abuse*. R. L. Dupont, A. Goldstein, and J. O'Donnell, eds. National Institute on Drug Abuse. US Government Printing Office, Washington, DC, pp. 3–16.

[4]M. D. Anglin (1988) (Special issue) A social policy analysis of compulsory treatment for opiate dependence, *J. Drug Issues* **18,** 503,504.

[5]W. H. McGlothlin, M. D. Anglin, and B. D. Wilson (1978) Narcotic addiction and crime. *Criminology* **16,** 293–315.

[6]M. D. Anglin and G. R. Speckart (1986) Narcotics use, property crime and dealing: Structural dynamics across the addiction career. *J. Quan. Criminology* **2,** 197–233.

[7]M. D. Anglin and G. R. Speckart (1988) Narcotics use and crime: A multisample, multimethod analysis. *Criminology* **26,** 197–233.

[8]M. D. Anglin and Y.-I. Hser (1987) Addicted women and crime. *Criminology* **25,** 359–397.

[9]J. C. Ball, E. Corty, H. R. Bond, and A. Tommasello (1987) The reduction of intravenous heroin use, non-opiate abuse and crime during methadone maintenance treatment-further findings. Paper presented at the annual meeting of the Committee on Problems of Drug Dependence, Philadelphia, June.

[10]H. J. Harwood, R. L. Hubbard, J. J. Collins, and J. V. Rachal (1988) The costs of crime and the benefits of drug abuse treatment: A cost-benefit analysis using TOPS data, in *Compulsory Treatment of Drug Abuse: Research and Clinical Practice* (NIDA Research Monograph 86). C. G. Leukefeld and F. M. Tims, eds. National Institute of Drug Abuse, Rockville, MD, pp. 209–235.

[11]R. L. Hubbard, M. Allison, R. M. Bray, S. G. Craddock, J. V. Rachal, and H. M. Ginzberg. (1983) An overview of client characteristics, treatment services, and during-treatment outcomes for outpatient prospective study (TOPS), in *Research on the Treatment of Narcotic Addiction: State of the Art* (NIDA Research Monograph 86). J. R. Cooper, F. Altman, B. S. Brown, and D. Czechowicz, eds. US Government Printing Office, Washington, DC, pp. 714–751.

[12]J. R. Cooper, F. Altman, B. S. Brown, and D. Czechowicz (eds.) (1983) *Research on the Treatment of Narcotics Addiction: State of the Art* (NIDA Research Monograph 86). National Institute on Drug Abuse, Rockville, MD.

[13]F. M. Tims and J. P. Ludford (eds.) (1984) *Drug Abuse Treatment Evaluation: Strategies, Process and Prospects* (NIDA Research Monograph 51). National Institute on Drug Abuse, Rockville, MD.

[14]J. C. Ball, L. Rosen, J. A. Flueck, and D. N. Nurco (1981) The criminality of heroin addicts when addicted and when off opiates, in *The Drugs–Crime Connection*. J. A. Inciardi, ed. Sage, Beverly Hills, CA, pp. 39–66.

[15]D. N. Nurco, J. W. Shaffer, J. C. Ball, and T. W. Kinlock (1984) Trends in the commission of crime among narcotic addicts over successive periods of addiction and nonaddiction. *Am. J. Drug Alcohol Abuse* **10,** 481–489.

[16]G. R. Speckart and M. D. Anglin (1986) Narcotics and crime: A causal modeling approach. *J. Quan. Criminology* **2,** 3–28.

[17]G. R. Speckart and M. D. Anglin (1986) Narcotics use and crime: An overview of recent research advances. *Contem. Drug Problems* **13,** 741–769.

[18]E. H. Adams, J. C. Gfroerer, B. A. Rouse, and N. J. Kozel (1987) Trends in prevalence and consequences of cocaine use. *Adv. Alcohol Subst. Abuse* **6,** 49–71.

[19]B. D. Johnson, P. Goldstein, E. Preble, J. Schmeidler, D. S. Lipton, B. Spunt, and T. Miller (1985) *Taking Care of Business: The Economics of Crime by Heroin Abusers.* Lexington Books, Lexington, MA.

[20]A. Goldstein, R. Norman, and B. Spunt (1982) Habitual criminal activity and patterns of drug use. Paper presented at the annual meeting of the American Society of Criminology, Toronto, Nov.

[21]D. N. Nurco, T. W. Kinlock, T. E. Hanlon, and J. C. Ball (1988) Nonnarcotic drug use over an addiction career—A study of heroin addicts in Baltimore and New York City. *Comp. Psychiatry* **29,** 450–459.

[22]M. D. Anglin, and Y.-I. Hser (1990) Treatment of drug abuse, in *Crime and Justice: An Annual Review of Research,* vol. 13. M. Tonry and J. Q. Wilson, eds. The University of Chicago Press, Chicago, pp. 393–460.

[23]National Association of State Alcohol and Drug Abuse Directors (NASAD) (1988) State Resources and Services Related to Alcohol and Drug Abuse Problems, Fiscal Year 1987.

[24]R. A. Rawson (1986) Inpatient treatment programs in the western United States. Unpublished manuscript. Los Angeles, CA.

[25]J. L. Sorenson, A. P. Acampora, M. Trier, and M. Gold (1987) From maintenance to abstinence in a therapeutic community: Follow-up outcomes. *J. Psychoactive Drugs* **19,** 345–351.

[26]B. J. Rounsaville (1989) Clinical assessment of drug abusers, in *Treatments of Psychiatric Disorders: A Task Force Report of the American Psychiatric Association,* vol. 2. H. Kleber, ed. American Psychiatric Association, Washington, D.C.

[27]J. C. Ball and E. Corty (1988) Basic issues pertaining to the effectiveness of methadone maintenance treatment, in *Compulsory Treatment of Drug Abuse: Research and Clinical Practice* (NIDA Research Monograph 86). C. G. Leukefeld and F. M. Tims, eds. National Institute on Drug Abuse, Rockville, MD, pp. 178–191.

[28]S. M. Hall (1984) Clinical trials in drug treatment: Methodology, in *Drug Abuse Treatment Evaluation: Strategies, Process and Prospects* (NIDA Research Monograph 51). F. Tims and J. Ludford, eds. National Institute on Drug Abuse, Rockville, MD, pp. 88–105.

[29]B. J. Rounsaville, T. Tierney, K. Crits-Christoph, M. M. Weissman, and H.

D. Kleber (1982) Predictors of outcome in treatment of opieate addict: Evidence for the multidimensional nature of addicts' problems. *Comp. Psychiatry* **23,** 462–478.

[30]R. L. Hubbard, J. V. Rachal, S. G. Craddock, and E. R. Cavanaugh (1984) Treatment outcome prospective study (TOPS): Client characteristics and behaviors before, during, and after treatment, in *Drug Abuse Treatment Evaluation: Strategies, Process and Prospects* (NIDA Research Monograph 51). F. Tims and J. Ludford, eds. National Institute on Drug Abuse, Rockville, MD.

[31]D. D. Simpson, L. J. Savage, M. R. Lloyd, and S. B. Sells (1978) *Evaluation of drug abuse treatments based on the first year after DARP: National follow-up study of admissions to drug abuse treatments in the DARP during 1969–1972* (NIDA Research Monograph). US Government Printing Office, Washington, DC.

[32]D. D. Simpson, and S. B. Sells (1982) *Evaluation of Drug Treatment Effectiveness: Summary of the DARP Follow-up Research* (NIDA Treatment Research Report). US Government Printing Office, Washington, DC.

[33]W. K. Bickel, I. Marion, and J. H. Lowinson (1987) The treatment of alcoholic methadone patients: A review. *J. Subst. Abuse Treatment* **4,** 15–19.

[34]E. Corty and J. C. Ball (1987) Admissions to methadone maintenance: Comparisons between programs and implications for treatment. *J. Subst. Abuse Treatment* **4,** 181–187.

[35]D. K. Roszell, D. A. Calsyn, and E. F. Chaney (1986) Alcohol use and psychopathology in opiod addicts on methadone maintenance. *Am. J. Drug Alcohol Abuse* **12,** 269–278.

[36]B. Stimmel, M. Cohen, and R. Hanbury (1978) Alcoholism and polydrug abuse in persons on methadone maintenance. *Ann. NY Acad. Sci.* **311,** 99–180.

[37]B. Stimmel, R. Hanbury, V. Sturiano, D. Korts, G. Jackson, and M. Cohen (1982) Alcoholism as a risk factor in methadone maintenence: A randomized controlled trial. *Am. J. Med.* **73,** 631–636.

[38]R. L. Hubbard, M. E. Marsden, E. Cavanaugh, J. V. Rachal, and H. M. Ginzburg (1988) Role of drug-abuse treatment in limiting the spread of AIDS. *Rev. Infectious Dis.* **10,** 377–384.

[39]M. A. Marcovici, T. McLellan, C. P. O'Brian, and J. Rosenzweig (1980) Risk for alcoholism and methadone treatment: A longitudinal study. *J. Nerv. Mental Disease* **168,** 556–558.

[40]R. L. Hubbard, M. E. Marsden, J. V. Rachal, H. J. Harwood, E. R. Cavanaugh, and H. M. Ginzberg (1989) *Drug Abuse Treatment: A National Study of Effectiveness.* University of North Carolina Press, Chapel Hill, NC.

[41]M. D. Anglin (1988) The efficacy of civil commitment in treating narcotics addiction. *J. Drug Issues* **18,** 527–546.

[42]D. A. Brizer, N. Hartman, J. Sweeney, and R. B. Millman (1985) Effect of methadone plus neuroleptics on treatment-resistant chronic paranoid

schizophrenia. *Am. J. Psychiatry* **142,** 1106,1107.

[43]H. D. Kleber (1986) The use of psychotropic drugs in the treatment of compulsive opiate abusers: The rationale for their use. *Adv. Alcohol Subst. Abuse* **5,** 103–119.

[44]A. T. McLellan, A. R. Childress, J. Griffith, and G. E. Woody (1984) The psychiatrically severe drug abuse patient: Methadone maintenance or therapeutic community. *Am. J. Drug Alcohol Abuse* **10,** 77–95.

[45]A. T. McLellan, L. Luborsky, G. E. Woody, C. P. O'Brian, and K. A. Druley (1983) Predicting response to alcohol and drug abuse treatments. *Arch. Gen. Psychiatry* **40,** 620–625.

[46]G. E. Woody, C. P. O'Brian, A. T. McLellan, and J. Mintz (1981) Psychotherapy for opiate addiction: Some preliminary results. *Ann. NY Acad. Sci.* **362,** 91–100.

[47]E. C. Senay (1984) Clinical implications of drug abuse treatment outcome research, in *Drug Abuse Treatment Evaluation: Strategies, Process and Prospects* (NIDA Research Monograph 51). F. Tims and J. Ludford, eds. National Institute on Drug Abuse, Rockville, MD, pp. 139–150.

[48]V. P. Dole and M. E. Nyswander (1965) A medical treatment of diacetylmorphine (heroin) addiction. *JAMA* **193,** 646–650.

[49]J. C. Ball, E. Corty, S. P. Petroski, H. Bond, and A. Tommasello (1986) Medical services provided to 2,394 patients at methadone programs in three states. *J. Subst. Abuse Treatment* **3,** 203–209.

[50]E. C. Senay (1985) Methadone maintenance treatment. *Int. J. Addict.* **20,** 803–821.

[51]Y.-I. Hser, M. D. Anglin, and C. Chou (1987) A repeated measures design for treatment evaluation. Paper presented at the annual meeting of American Educational Research Association, Washington, DC.

[52]M. D. Anglin and W. H. McGlothlin (1985) Methadone maintenance in California: A decade's experience, in *The Yearbook of Substance Use and Abuse.* L. Brill and C. Winick, eds. Human Sciences Press, New York.

[53]M. D. Anglin and W. H. McGlothlin (1984) Outcome of narcotic addict treatment in California, in *Drug Abuse Treatment Evaluation: Strategies, Process and Prospects* (NIDA Research Monograph 51). F. Tims and J. Ludford, eds. National Institute on Drug Abuse, Rockville, MD.

[54]J. F. Maddux and D. P. Desmond (1979) Crime and drug use behavior: An areal analysis. *Criminology* **19,** 281–302.

[55]A. T. McLellan, L. Luborsky, C. P. O'Brian, G. E. Woody, and K. A. Druley (1982) Is treatment for substance abuse effective? *JAMA* **247,** 1423–1428.

[56]Burt Associates, Inc. (1977) *Drug Treatment in New York City and Washington, D.C.: Follow-up Studies.* US Government Printing Office, Washington, DC.

[57]W. H. McGlothlin and M. D. Anglin (1981) Shutting off methadone: Costs and benefits. *Arch. Gen. Psychiatry* **38,** 885–892.

[58]M. D. Anglin, G. R. Speckart, M. W. Booth, and T. M. Ryan (1989) Consequences and costs of shutting off methadone. *Addict. Behav.* **14,** 307–326.

[59]W. H. McGlothlin and M. D. Anglin (1981) Long-term follow-up of clients of high- and low-dose methadone programs. *Arch. Gen. Psychiatry* **38,** 1055–1063.

[60]D. G. Fisher and M. D. Anglin (1987) Survival analysis in drug program evaluation: Part I. Overall program effectiveness. *Int. J. Addict.* **22,** 115–134.

[61]M. Stitzer (1977) Medication take-home as a reinforcer in a methadone maintenance program. *Addict. Behav.* **2,** 9–14.

[62]J. B. Milby, C. Garrett, C. English, O. Fritshi, and C. Clark (1978) Take-home methadone: Contingency effects on drug-seeking and productivity of narcotic addicts. *Addict. Behav.* **3,** 215–220.

[63]M. Stitzer, G. E. Bigelow, and J. Gross (1989) Behavioral treatment of drug abuse, in *Treatments of Psychiatric Disorders: A Task Force Report of the American Psychiatric Association,* vol. 2. H. Kleber, ed. American Psychiatric Association, Washington, DC.

[64]D. V. Biase (1981) Daytop miniversity: Advancement in drug-free therapeutic community treatment. Evaluation Report No. 1-H81-DA-01911-0A1. National Institute on Drug Abuse, Rockville, MD.

[65]G. De Leon (1985) The therapeutic community: Status and evolution. *Int. J. Addict.* **20,** 823–844.

[66]S. B. Sells ed. (1974) *Evaluation of Treatment,* vols. 1,2. Ballinger, Cambridge, MA.

[67]G. De Leon (1984) Program-based evaluation research in therapeutic communities, in *Drug Abuse Treatment Evaluation: Strategies, Process and Prospects* (NIDA Research Monograph 51). National Institute on Drug Abuse, Rockville, MD, pp. 69–87.

[68]W. S. Aron and D. W. Daily (1976) Graduates and splittees from therapeutic community drug treatment programs: A comparison. *Int. J. Addict.* **11,** 1–18.

[69]H. Barr and D. Antes (1981) *Factors Related to Recovery and Relapse in Followup.* Final Report of Project Activities, Grant No. l-H81-DA-01864. National Institute on Drug Abuse, Rockville, MD.

[70]R. C. Brook and I. C. Whitehead (1980) *Drug-Free Therapeutic Community.* Human Sciences Press, New York.

[71]De Leon, G., M. P. A. Andrews, H. K. Weer, J. Jaffe, and M. S. Rosenthal (1979) Therapeutic community dropouts: Criminal behavior five years after treatment. *Am. J. Drug Alcohol Abuse* **6,** 253–271.

[72]S. Holland (1978) Gateway houses: Effectiveness of treatment on criminal behavior. *Int. J. Addict.* **13,** 369–381.

[73]S. Holland (1983) Evaluating community-based treatment programs: A

model for strengthening inferences about effectiveness. *Int. J. Ther. Community* **4,** 285–306.

[74]E. J. Pin, J. M. Martine, and J. F. Walsh (1976) A follow-up study of 300 ex-clients of a drug-free narcotic treatment program in New York City. *Am. J. Drug Alcohol Abuse* **3,** 397–407.

[75]K. F. Pompi, S. C. Shreiner, and J. L. McKey (1979) *Abraxas: A First Look at Outcomes.* Abraxas Foundation, Pittsburgh, PA.

[76]A. M. Romond, C. K. Forrest, and H. D. Kleber (1975) Follow-up of participants in a drug dependence therapeutic community. *Arch. Gen. Psychiatry* **32,** 369–374.

[77]S. R. Wilson (1978) The effect of treatment in a therapeutic community on intravenous drug abuse. *J. Addict.* **73,** 407–411.

[78]S. R. Wilson and B. M. Mandelbrote (1978) The relationship between duration of treatment in a therapeutic community for drug abusers and subsequent criminality. *J. Med. Psychol.* **132,** 487–491.

[79]R. H. Coombs (1981) Back on the streets: Therapeutic communities' impact upon drug abusers. *Am. J. Alcohol Abuse* **8,** 185–201.

[80]G. De Leon (1983) *The T.C.: Predicting Retention and Followup Status.* Final Report No. 1-ROl-DA-02741-01Al. National Institute on Drug Abuse, Washington, DC.

[81]G. De Leon (1983) The therapeutic community approach to rehabilitation: Perspective and a study of effectiveness, in *Drug and Alcohol Use Issues and Factors.* S. Einstein, ed. Plenum, New York.

[82]G. De Leon, A. Skodol, and M. S. Rosenthal (1973) The Phoenix therapeutic community for drug addicts: Changes in psychopathological signs. *Arch. Gen. Psychiatry* **23,** 131–135.

[83]R. A. Rawson, J. L. Obert, and M. J. McCann (1990) The treatment of cocaine addiction and alcoholism at Sierra Tucson: Treatment outcome issues. Unpublished manuscript.

[84]R. N. Bale, W. W. Van Stone, J. M. Kuldau, T. J. M. Engelsing, R. M. Elashoff, and V. P. Zarcone (1980) Therapeutic communities vs methadone maintenance: A prospective controlled study of narcotic addiction treatment. *Arch. Gen. Psychiatry* **37,** 179–193.

[85]D. D. Simpson (1984) National treatment system evaluation based on the drug abuse reporting program (DARP) follow-up research, in *Drug Abuse Treatment Evaluation: Strategies, Process and Prospects* (NIDA Research Monograph 51). National Institute on Drug Abuse, Rockville, MD.

[86]E. D. Wish (1987) National Institute of Justice drug use forecasting: New York 1984–1986, in *National Institute of Justice Research in Action.* The Department of Justice, Washington, DC.

[87]C. A. Innes (1988) Bureau of Justice Statistics, *Drug Use and Crime.* Washington, DC.

[88]D. Lipton, R. Martinson, and J. Wilks (1975) *The Effectiveness of Correctional Treatment: A Survey of Treatment Evaluation Studies.* Praeger, New York.

[89]G. M. Camp and C. G. Camp (1989) *Building on Prior Experiences: Therapeutic Communities in Prisons.* Criminal Justice Institute, South Salem, NY.

[90]R. C. Newman (1980) Diversion of Addicts from the Criminal Justice System to Treatment. National Conference on Standards, Ethics and Practice. New York University/Bellvue Forensic Psychiatry Service.

[91]M. W. Klein (1979) Deinstitutionalization and diversion of juvenile offenders: A litany of impediments, in *Crime and Justice: An Annual Review of Research.* vol. 1. N. Morris and M. Tonry, eds. University of Chicago Press, Chicago, IL, pp. 145–201.

[92]B. J. Bullington, D. K. Sprowls, and M. Phillips (1978) A critique of "diversionary juvenile justice." *Crime Delinquency* **24,** 59–71.

[93]F. Allen (1959) Criminal justice, legal values, and the rehabilitative ideal. *J. Criminal Law, Criminology, Police Sci.* **50,** 226–232.

[94]S. Cohen (1979) The punitive city: Notes on the dispersal of society control. *Contemp. Crisis* **3,** 339–363.

[95]R. W. Salmon and R. J. Salmon (1983) The role of coercion in rehabilitation of drug abusers. *Int. J. Addict.* **18,** 9–21.

[96]T. Orsagh and M. E. Marsden (1985) What works when: Rational-choice theory and offender rehabilitation. *J. Criminal Justice* **13,** 269–277.

[97]M. D. Anglin and Y.-I. Hser (1990) Legal coercion and drug abuse treatment: Research findings and social policy implications, in *Handbook of Drug Control in the United States.* J. Inciardi, ed. Greenwood Press, Westport, CT, pp. 151–176.

[98]W. H. McGlothlin, M. D. Anglin, and B. D. Wilson (1977) *An Evaluation of the California Civil Addict Program.* Services Research Issues Series. National Institute on Drug Abuse, Rockville, MD.

[99]M. D. Anglin and W. H. McGlothlin (1985) Methadone maintenance in California: A decade's experience, in *The Yearbook of Substance Use and Abuse.* L. Brill and C. Winick, eds. Human Sciences Press, New York, pp. 219–280.

[100]C. S. Winick (1962) Maturing out of narcotic addiction. *Bull. Narc.* **14,** 1–7.

[101]H. K. Wexler, D. S. Lipton, and K. Foster (1985) Outcome evaluation of a prison therapeutic community for substance abuse treatment: Preliminary results. Paper presented at the American Society of Criminology Annual Meeting, San Diego, November.

[102]D. A. Andrews, I. Zinger, R. D. Hoge, J. Bonta, P. Gendreau, and F. T. Cullen (in press) Does correctional treatment work? A clinically relevant and psychologically informed meta-analysis. *Criminology.*

[103]L. F. Cook, B. A. Weinman et al. (1988) Treatment alternatives to street crime, in *Compulsory Treatment of Drug Abuse: Research and Clinical Practice* (NIDA Research Monograph 86). C. G. Leukefeld and F. M. Tims, eds. National

Institute on Drug Abuse, Rockville, MD, pp. 99–105.

[104]S. B. Sells (1984) Drug abuse treatment effectiveness—reduction of drug-related offenses among opiate addicts, in *Encyclopedia of Crime and Justice*, vol. 2, S. H. Kadish, ed. Free Press, New York.

[105]J. J. Collins and M. Allison (1983) Legal coercion and retention in drug abuse treatment. *Hospital Community Psychiatry* **34,** 1145–1149.

[106]R. A. McFarlain, G. H. Cohen, J. Yoder, and L. Guidry (1977) Psychological test and demographic variables associated with retention of narcotics addicts in treatment. *Int. J. Addict.* **12,** 399–410.

[107]S. H. Schnoll, M. R. Goldstein, D. E. Antes, and V. J. Rinella (1980) The impact of legal involvement on substance abusers in a residential treatment setting. *Corrective Soc. Psychiatry J. Behav. Technol. Methods, Ther.* **26,** *21–28.*

[108]S. B. Sells and D. D. Simpson (eds.) (1976) *The Effectiveness of Drug Abuse Treatment: vol. 3 Further Studies of Drug Users, Treatment Typologies, and Assessments of Outcomes During Treatment in the DARP.* Ballinger, Cambridge, MA.

[109]S. B. Sells and D. D. Simpson (eds.) (1976) *The Effectiveness of Drug Abuse Treatment: vol. 4 Evaluation of Treatment Outcomes for 1971–1972 DARP Admission Cohort.* Ballinger, Cambridge, MA.

[110]S. B. Sells and D. D. Simpson (eds.) (1976) *The Effectiveness of Drug Abuse Treatment: vol. 5 Evaluation of Treatment Outcomes for 1972–1973 DARP Admission Cohort.* Ballinger, Cambridge, MA.

[111]D. D. Simpson and J. Friend (1988) Legal status and long-term outcomes for addicts in the DARP follow-up project, in *Compulsory Treatment of Drug Abuse: Research and Clinical Practice* (NIDA Research Monograph 86). C. G. Leukefeld and F. M. Tims, eds. National Institute on Drug Abuse, Rockville, MD, pp. 81–98.

[112]M. D. Anglin, M. L. Brecht, and E. Maddahian (1990) Pre-treatment characteristics and treatment performance of legally coerced versus voluntary methadone maintenance admissions. *Criminology* **27,** 537–557.

[113]M. D. Anglin and K. I. Powers (1991) Individual and joint effects of methadone maintenance and legal supervision on the behavior of narcotics addicts, in press.

[114]H. J. Harwood, R. L. Hubbard, J. J. Collins, and J. V. Rachal (1988) The costs of crime and the benefits of drug abuse treatment: A cost-benefit analysis using TOPS data, in *Compulsory Treatment of Drug Abuse: Research and Clinical Practice* (NIDA Research Monograph 86). C. G. Leukefeld and F. M. Tims, eds. National Institute on Drug Abuse, Rockville, MD, pp. 209–235.

[115]D. P. Rice, S. Kelman, and S. Dunmeyer (1990) *The Economic Costs of Alcohol and Drug Abuse and Mental Illness: 1985.* Report submitted to the Office of Financing and Coverage Policy of the Alcohol, Drug Abuse, and Mental Health Administration, US Department of Health and Human Services. DHHS Pub.

No. (ADM)90-1694. Institute of Health and Aging, University of California, San Diego.

[116]S. S. Wallack (1990) Cost of Drug Abuse Treatments. Testimony to the legislation and national security subcommittee of the House Government Operations Committee. April 17.

[117]B. T. Yates (1985) Cost-effectiveness analysis and cost-benefit analysis: An introduction. *Behav. Assess.* **7,** 207–234.

[118]W. A. Hargreaves (1983) Methadone dose and duration for maintenance treatment: Methodology, in *Research on the Treatment of Narcotics Addiction: State of the Art* (NIDA Research Monograph). J. R. Cooper, F. Altman, B. S. Brown, and D. Czechowicz, eds. National Institute on Drug Abuse, Rockville, MD.

[119]G. W. Joe, D. D. Simpson, and S. B. Sells (1992) Treatment process and relapse to opioid use during methadone maintenance. *Am. J. Alcohol Drug Abuse* (in press).

[120]C. P. O'Brian, A. R. Childress, A. T. McLellan, J. Ternes, and R. N. Ehrman (1984) Use of naltrexone to extinguish opioid-conditioned responses. *J. Clin. Psychiatry* **45,** 53.

[121]B. J. Rounsaville, W. Glazer, C. H. Wilber, M. M. Weissman, and H. D. Kleber (1983) Short-term interpersonal psychotherapy in methadone maintained opiate addicts. *Arch. Gen. Psychiatry* **40,** 629–636.

[122]G. E. Woody, L. Luborsky, A. T. McLellan, and J. Mintz (1983) Psychotherapy for opiate addicts: Does it help? *Arch. Gen. Psychiatry* **40,** 639–645.

[123]E. Wish and B. Gropper (1990) Drug testing by the criminal justice system: Methods, research, and applications, in *Drugs and Crime*, vol. 13. M. Tonry and J. Q. Wilson, eds. University of Chicago Press, Chicago, IL, pp. 321–391.

[124]M. D. Anglin, E. P. Deschenes, and G. R. Speckart (1987) The effect of legal supervision on narcotic addiction and criminal behavior. Paper presented at the annual meeting of the American Society of Criminology, Montreal, November.

[125]G. R. Speckart, M. D. Anglin, and E. P. Deschenes (1989) Modeling the longitudinal impact of legal sanctions on narcotics use and property crime. *J. Quan. Criminology*, **5,** 35–36.

[126]W. H. McGlothin and M. D. Anglin (1979) Effects of closing the Bakersfield methadone clinic, in *Problems of Drug Dependence: 1979* (NIDA Research Monograph 47). L. S. Harris, ed. National Institute on Drug Abuse, Rockville, MD, pp. 135–141.

[127]D. D. Simpson (1979) The relation of time spent in drug-abuse treatment to post-treatment outcome. *Am. J. Psychiatry* **136,** 1449–1453.

[128]D. D. Simpson (1984) Treatment for drug abuse: Follow-up outcomes and length of time spent. *Arch. Gen. Psychiatry* **38,** 875–880.

[129]G. De Leon and S. Schwartz (1984) The therapeutic community: What are the retention rates? *J. Drug Alcohol Abuse* **10,** 267–284.

[130]J. F. Maddux and C. L. Bowden (1972) Critique of success with methadone

maintenance. *Am. J. Psychiatry* **129,** 440–446.

[131]F. Baekland and L. Lundwall (1975) Dropping out of treatment: A critical review. *Psychol. Bull.* **82,** 738–783.

[132]H. K. Wexler and G. De Leon (1977) The therapeutic community: Multivariate prediction of retention. *Am. J. Drug Alcohol Abuse* **4,** 145–151.

[133]R. A. Steer (1980) Psychosocial correlates of retention in methadone maintenance. *Int. J. Addict.* **15,** 1003–1009.

[134]A. T. McLellan, G. E. Woody, B. Evans, and C. P. O'Brian (1989) Methadone vs. therapeutic community in the treatment of mixed abusers: Role of psychiatic symptoms. *Ann. NY Acad. Sci.* (forthcoming).

[135]J. Sansone (1980) Retention patterns in a therapeutic community for the treatment of drug abuse. *Int. J. Addict.* **15,** 711–736.

[136]G. De Leon (1987) Alcohol use among drug abusers: Treatment outcomes in a therapeutic community. *Alcohol. Clin. Exp. Res.* **11,** 430–436.

[137]S. B. De Leon and D. D. Simpson (eds.) (1976) *The Effectiveness of Drug Abuse Treatment,* vols. 3–5. Ballinger, Cambridge, MA.

[138]J. C. Ball and A. Ross (eds.) (1991) *The Effectiveness of Methadone Maintenance Treatment: Patients, Programs, Services & Outcome.* Springer-Verlag, New York.

[139]C. D. D'Amanda (1983) Program policies and procedures associated with treatment outcome, in *Research on the Treatment of Narcotics Addiction: State of the Art* (NIDA Research Monograph). J. R. Cooper, F. Altman, B. S. Brown, and D. Czechowicz, eds. National Institute on Drug Abuse, Rockville, MD.

[140]L. Wermuth, S. Brummett, and J. L. Sorenson (1987) Bridges and barriers to recovery: Clinical observations from an opiate-recovery project. *J. Subst. Abuse Treatment* **4,** 189–196.

The Organization and Impact of Outpatient Drug Abuse Treatment Services

Richard H. Price
and Thomas A. D'Aunno

Evolution of the Drug Abuse Treatment Service in the US

Conceptions of Drug Abuse in the US

Gerstein and Harwood[1] observed that our national response to drug abuse has historically been governed by simple, but powerful ideas. From the time of the Revolution to the Reconstruction period, drug abuse was considered private behavior and a *libertarian* view prevailed. The late 1800s saw the emergence of a *medical* conception, and treatments, including detoxification, developed. Early in this century, a *criminal* conception developed, and drug control became the characteristic response.

Today, each of these ideas has some influence on the organization of services. There has been a reemergence of the medical view as well as the idea that treatment is a public good and should, in principle, be available to all. In the 1980s, support for the public sector has not kept up with demand, and a private-for-profit drug treatment sector has grown. At the same time, public responsibility for treatment has shifted from the federal government to the states.

From: *Drug and Alcohol Abuse Reviews, Vol. 4: Drug Abuse Treatment*
Ed: R. R. Watson

It is in the context of this complex picture of shifting ideas about drug treatment, changing funding patterns, and shifting responsibility between public and private sectors and federal and state government that drug abuse treatment services are best understood. In the following chapter, we examine recent developments and discuss program factors that affect those seeking treatment, retention in treatment, and efficacy. We also concern ourselves with special populations, high-risk groups, and important treatment modalities, such as methadone treatment. The recurring theme of this chapter is that organizational policy issues importantly shape access to care and its effectiveness. Furthermore, there is frequently a gap between what is known about effective treatment and the way treatment is actually delivered in the field. This chapter notes these gaps whenever possible.

Recent Developments in the Drug Abuse Treatment System

The nation's system of outpatient treatment for drug abuse is undergoing large systematic changes that have important implications for the organization and effectiveness of outpatient drug abuse treatment. The movement of outpatient drug abuse treatment services into the mental health sector and the health care system in general,[2] and the shift of drug abuse treatment from federal to state control[3] both are major changes in the environment influencing services in ways that may ultimately shape treatment efficiency and effectiveness.[4]

In addition, new kinds of clients are being served by the outpatient drug abuse treatment system, which presents that system with new challenges. Jaffee[5] and Frances[6] have observed that a substantial proportion of drug abuse patients show signs of depression or psychopathology. The question can be asked, "Will drug abuse treatment delivered in the mental health system or in other systems be more responsive to multiproblem patients with both drug abuse and mental health problems, or will one set of problems receive undue attention at the expense of the other?"

In addition, the Omnibus Reconciliation Act of 1981 dramatically changed the way in which federal support is provided for drug abuse treatment. The Act provided that alcohol, drug abuse, and mental health block grants be administered by the individual states rather than by the National Institute on Drug Abuse.[3] The shift to state authority may provide the opportunity for better coordination of outpatient treatment at the state level or may increase fragmentation of treatment services.

All of these changes suggest that the degree to which services are meeting the needs of clients, the availability of special treatment modalities, such as outpatient methadone treatment, and the availability of services for special populations are critical issues facing the national drug abuse service system. This chapter addresses these issues. It also addresses questions concerning the degree to which ownership and financing differences affect the type of clients served and the range of services available in the outpatient drug abuse treatment system.

Client and Program Factors That Affect Treatment Seeking, Retention, and Treatment Efficacy

Client Characteristics

The demographic and social background of clients in substance abuse programs is a critical ingredient in understanding client and program factors that affect treatment seeking, retention, and efficacy. The results of the National Outpatient Drug Abuse Treatment System Survey[7] indicate that across the entire outpatient drug treatment system, respondents reported that 54% of their clients had multiple drug problems. Furthermore, 41% of outpatient clients were reported to have marijuana problems, 27% cocaine problems, 24% heroin problems, 13% crack abuse problems, and 13% tranquilizer abuse problems. Finally, approx half of clients in this sample had alcohol problems as their primary difficulty.

Comparing drug-free and methadone programs provided some striking contrasts. Methadone programs tended to have markedly fewer clients where alcohol was the primary problem, more heroin problems, and more problems with nonprescription methadone, cocaine, and tranquilizers, but fewer clients with amphetamine or LSD problems. More methadone clients also tested positive or were diagnosed to have AIDS, especially in hospital treatment settings. On the other hand, mental health centers tended to have fewer clients whose primary problem was drug abuse. Overall, survey data on client demographics indicated that two-thirds of the clients being served were male, 11% Hispanic, and 19% Black. The age distribution of clients is primarily young, with 78% of the sample being 39 yr or younger. Clients in methadone programs tended to be older and were more likely to be Hispanic or Black.

Staffing Patterns

On the average, outpatient treatment units in this national sample tended to be fairly small, with about 13 treatment staff members in methadone units and about nine on the average in drug-free units. In methadone units, staff tended to have medical training, especially as nurses and physicians. Methadone units tended to have fewer Ph.D.s and fewer Masters level staff, and also to have fewer staff with substance abuse treatment certification or training when compared with drug-free programs.

Staffing patterns also differed according to the type of organization in which the treatment unit was embedded. Mental health centers tended to have the most highly educated staff with the most months of substance abuse training. Mental health centers also tended to have fewer exaddicts as staff members. Treatment units that were either free-standing or embedded in human service organizations other than hospitals and mental health centers tended in general to have lower levels of educational qualifications among their staff and to have more part-time staff.

Medical and Social Services Provided in Outpatient Drug Abuse Treatment

One of the most prominent characteristics of chronic drug abusers is that they suffer from a variety of serious health and social problems, including unemployment, poor family relations, and mental health problems. Accordingly, it is widely agreed that to be successful, treatment programs must assess a variety of client needs and provide services to meet those needs effectively.[8,9] For example, the Addiction Severity Index[10] was developed specifically to assess six client needs: drug use, psychological problems, family problems, vocational adjustment, legal problems, and medical problems.

Of these problem areas, researchers have given most attention to mental health problems and services in drug abuse treatment.[11-13] Data from the Treatment Outcome Prospective Study (TOPS)[14] indicate that drug abuse clients have a great need for mental health services. Of the 10,000 clients who participated in TOPS, 60% reported some symptom of depression in the year before admission. Further, the weight of the evidence indicates that the addition of psychotherapy to drug abuse treatment counseling improves treatment outcomes for methadone clients.[13] Other services, though less well examined, are also important. For example, a recent study of 590 methadone clients and 21 treatment clients who participated in TOPS[15] found that relapse to opioid use was less likely for clients who had more ancillary services, particularly mental health, employment, and general services.

Despite the widely held belief in the importance of assessing and meeting the many needs of drug abusers in treatment, we know very little about the medical and social services provided by drug abuse treatment units. Most studies of such services rely on small, limited samples of units, and, as a result, it is difficult to draw meaningful conclusions about the provision of such services across the nation. Thus, results from the National Outpatient Drug Abuse Treatment System Survey are particularly important, because this study draws data from a national random sample of 575 treatment units.

The results of the study have important implications for policymakers and administrators concerned with planning and providing services for outpatient drug abuse treatment clients. First, the results suggest that units are not providing enough of certain services, especially mental health care and financial and employment counseling, to meet clients' needs. Data from the TOPS study[8] indicate that 44–62% of all outpatient clients reported having financial problems. The national survey data indicate that on the average, only 27% of clients receive financial counseling.

Similarly, TOPS data show that mental health problems were cited by 33–50% of outpatient clients. The national survey data indicate that on the average, only 36% of clients are receiving mental health care from their treatment units. This gap is especially significant given the results from previous studies that indicate that mental health treatment increases the effectiveness of drug abuse treatment, particularly for methadone clients.[13,15]

TOPS data also show that approx 20–30% of clients were not involved in productive activity immediately before entering treatment. Only about 25% of the clients in the TOPS study were fully employed (40 wk or more) in the year before they entered treatment. The national survey data indicate that one-third of all clients, on the average, are receiving employment counseling. Thus, more than one-third of clients in treatment may need or benefit from employment counseling.

In contrast, units may be meeting the medical care needs of clients somewhat better. TOPS data show that medical problems were least frequently cited by outpatient clients (about one-third), and the national survey data indicate that about 38% of outpatient clients are receiving medical care from their drug abuse treatment units.

A second major conclusion from this study is that substantial variation in the provision of medical and social services is accounted for by client and unit characteristics. Units that treat more Black and heroin clients tend to provide more services for clients. These findings raise a key question: Is this level and distribution of services adequate? Future research should be directed at understanding why there are differences among client groups in the amount and type of medical and social services received in drug abuse treatment. Are such differences related to the need for services or other factors?

The results indicate that units are more likely to provide medical care when they are affiliated with hospitals, and when they have broad treatment goals and more staff members. Similarly, units are more likely to provide mental health care when they are affiliated with hospitals, and when they have broad treatment goals and more professional staff members.

Hospital affiliation may be important, because it links units and their clients to professionals and services that are otherwise difficult to access.[16] That is, hospitals typically have medical and mental health professionals on staff who would be available to provide services for the clients of the hospital's drug abuse treatment units. In fact, some hospitals have diversified into drug abuse treatment in order to offset the loss of patients in their traditional services.[17] Drug abuse clients may be benefiting from such diversification with increased access to medical and mental health care.

Finally, the breadth of treatment goals is the most important unit characteristic in service provision. Units that have broad goals are likely to provide more services to clients. This finding may have important implications for administrators who view their unit's mission narrowly. That is, many administrators should focus more attention on the spectrum of client needs and define their unit's mission accordingly. A broader definition of mission does not necessarily mean that units should provide a range of services themselves. Rather, broader treatment goals can be met first by conducting adequate assessments of a range of client needs (using, for example, the Addiction Severity Index) and, second, by making effective referrals to other service providers. The chief limitation of making such referrals is that too often drug abuse clients "fall through the cracks" and never reach other service providers. Nonetheless, a referral network may be the best service that many drug abuse treatment units can provide for their clients given limited resources.

Correlates of Effectiveness in the Drug-Free Outpatient System

A large number of clinical studies have been conducted with the goal of identifying those aspects of drug abuse and alcohol treatment services that produce effective results. Most of the studies of this kind have been small-scale, nonrandomized trials in which clients participating in different forms of treatment are followed over time. A large number of different aspects of treatment services has been identified as potentially important in ensuring treatment effectiveness. However, most of these clinical trials have had research design problems that render the results reported equivocal. We begin by briefly reviewing those clinical trials that randomly assigned clients to various aspects of treatment or control groups. Although this represents a much smaller number of studies, it is more likely that the results reported can be relied upon.

At least two randomized studies have attempted to understand the interaction between the type of client treated and the treatment program. For example, one study[18] compared drug therapy, psychotherapy plus drug therapy, and inpatient individual therapy with a control group in a randomized trial involving 458 adults. The results were complex, with different social and psychological factors of individuals doing better with different treatment program types. A second study[19] examined the interaction of treatment client type with treatment program in a prison-based program comparing group therapy with routine institutional care only. In a 1-yr follow-up, the researchers found that group therapy failed to produce lower recidivism rates than routine institutional care. However, different types of offenders experienced different rates of success with different types of treatments.

A second type of randomized trial has tended to measure treatment intensity as a major dimension by comparing minimal treatment with more intensive and elaborate programs. For example, Miller et al.[20] used focused vs broad spectrum behavior therapy as the treatment of interest. They randomly assigned 56 adults to self-help, behavioral self-control, or behavioral self-control plus various programs teaching specific coping skills. They found no significant difference in effectiveness between minimal patient treatment training and more extensive interventions. Miller et al. also noted that there was a strong positive relationship between therapist's skill, particularly showing empathy, and successful client outcomes. A second study of this type focused on coping skills and relaxation training, beginning with a randomized assignment to either minimal treatment or minimal treatment plus various specific training programs for coping skills. The follow-up 30-d after treatment completion indicated that all treatment modes improved clinical outcomes, and no differences in outcomes were observed by treatment mode.

Still other aspects of treatment involve the use of prescription drugs in treatment. Fuller et al.[21] studied disulfiram treatment for alcoholism in a randomized control trial with 605 adult males. They found that disulfiram may help reduce drinking frequency after relapse, but it does not enhance counseling in aiding patients to sustain abstinence or delay the resumption of drinking.

Finally, Gilbert[22] examined the effectiveness of aftercare on various treatment outcomes in a randomized trial with 96 male VA patients. Gilbert found that appointment-keeping significantly improved with home visit aftercare, and home visit aftercare increased the probability of treatment completion, but did not affect the number of hospital days during 1-yr follow-up.

Much of the research just reported is limited in a number of important ways. Much of it is based on findings from small samples of clients or drug treatment units of unknown representativeness. In addition, few studies of the characteristics of an effective treatment program have used multivariate analyses and adequate controls to account for variation in outcomes owing to client characteristics. Third, outcomes may depend on aspects of treatment that occur at a particular stage in the course of the client's treatment career, such as during diagnosis or aftercare. Few studies have differentiated treatment characteristics according to the stage of treatment. Finally, much of the research on components of effective treatment has focused on inpatient residential treatment. However, recent studies suggest that outpatient drug treatment may be just as high in quality as inpatient treatment.[23]

A recent study by McCaughrin and Price[24] used survey data from a national survey of outpatient drug abuse treatment units conducted in 1988 by the University of Michigan's Institute for Social Research. The sample of treatment units for the national study conducted by McCaughrin and Price focused on outpatient nonmethadone drug treatment units only. The sample size was 394. They focused on two major measures of treatment effectiveness: first, the percentage of clients who were reported to have met goals set for their treatment among clients who ended treatment in the last fiscal year, and second, the percentage of clients who were reported to continue to misuse drugs or alcohol. A number of control variables were included in the analyses conducted by McCaughrin and Price to rule out the possibility that outcomes were the result of the characteristics of the clients themselves, organizational characteristics of the treatment units themselves, and social area characteristics of the geographical area in which the treatment occurred. In addition, variables were identified at various stages of the treatment program, including referral into the program, assessment and diagnosis, various aspects of treatment, and posttreatment and follow-up stages of treatment. Similar findings were obtained for program characteristics predicting both measures of treatment effectiveness. In particular, follow-up efforts appear to be a promising characteristic of effective treatment programs and more favorable client–staff ratios were associated with better outcomes.

McCaughrin and Price also found that units with formal written quality assurance plans had higher percentages of clients who continued to misuse drugs and alcohol. This finding appears paradoxical, but may indicate a "discovery effect" created by the assurance plan. That is, a formal plan calls for careful surveillance and documentation of clients' progress during treatment, which could reveal empirical evidence of client recidivism that otherwise might not be observed.

It is interesting to observe that aftercare is a key element of effective treatment, as measured by both the randomized trials reviewed at the beginning of this section and in our National Outpatient Drug Abuse Treatment Survey results. In addition, it is interesting to note that some efforts to improve treatment quality, such as the development of quality assurance practices, may actually uncover cases of recidivism that might not otherwise have been noted.

Variation in Methadone Treatment Practices

The use of methadone to treat narcotic addiction continues to be controversial. Indeed, there is disagreement about several aspects of methadone maintenance treatment, including its overall effectiveness,[25] appropriate treatment goals (i.e., maintenance vs abstinence),[9] how to evaluate treatment programs,[26] effective dose levels,[27,28] the role of the government in regulating treatment policies and practices,[29] monitoring client behavior in treatment,[30,31] and the use of methadone maintenance to prevent HIV infection among needle-users.[32]

At the same time, however, there is an emerging consensus about two issues. First, methadone treatment for narcotic intravenous (iv) drug users is an important approach for preventing transmission of the human immunodeficiency virus (HIV).[9,33–37] Second, the longer clients remain in treatment, the less likely they are to return to illicit drug use and injections.[9,38–41] In turn, relatively high-dose treatment that includes client participation in dose decisions is related to higher retention rates.[28,41–43] In short, the weight of current evidence suggests that methadone treatment units that restrict dose levels and client participation in dose decisions are counterproductive both for reducing illicit drug use and for preventing HIV infection among narcotic needle-users.

D'Aunno and Vaughn[44] recently examined the extent to which a national random sample of outpatient methadone treatment units are engaging in restrictive treatment practices. They focused on several important treatment practices, including dose levels, client influence in and awareness of dose levels, take-home policies, and time limits set on detoxification. Further, they examined the relationship of these treatment practices to client time in treatment, which, as previously noted, is one of the most important factors in treatment effectiveness. Though some studies[9] have reported variation in treatment practices, there has not been a recent comprehensive study that provides policymakers and practitioners with an assessment of practices in the nation's outpatient methadone treatment system. Their study used data from a national survey of outpatient methadone treatment units conducted in the Fall of 1988 by the University of Michigan's Institute for Social Research (ISR).

The results indicate that there is substantial variation in the treatment practices of methadone maintenance units across the nation. The majority of units (66%) report that their clients are aware of their methadone dose level to a great or very great extent, but 34% of the units report that their clients are aware of their dose levels only to some, little, or no extent.

Similarly, units vary in the extent to which their clients influence dose levels and the extent to which they permit take-home dosages. In most units (56%), clients influence dose levels to some, little, or no extent; in contrast, 44% of the units report that clients influence dose levels to a great or very great extent. Most units (55%) permit take-home dosages to some, little, or no extent, but 47% of the units permit take-home dosages to a great or very great extent.

Further, the data indicate that units vary substantially in the dose levels they dispense. Twenty-five percent of the units typically set an upper limit on dose levels of 20–60 mg/d. In contrast, 30% of the units have an upper dose limit in excess of 80 mg/d.

The average dose level for the majority of the units (68%) is 50 mg/d or less, with 34% of the units reporting an average dose level of 40 mg/d or less. The data concerning dose levels indicate that most units (72%) have a balance between clients who are increasing and decreasing their dose levels. The remaining units, however, have more clients decreasing rather than increasing their dose levels, suggesting an emphasis on detoxification from methadone.

The data also show that 50% of the units encourage clients to detoxify in less than 6 mo. In contrast, 25% of the units do not encourage clients to detoxify until they have spent at least 12 mo in treatment. Finally, the data indicate that most units (54%) have an average length of client treatment of 20 mo or less.

It is important to point out that thousands of clients are affected by the treatment practices just reported. Specifically, these units reported treating nearly 34,000 clients in the previous year. Based on the number of clients treated at each unit, this means, for example, that 18,245 clients had only some, little, or no influence over their dose levels. Further, 7004 clients had average dose levels that most researchers consider too low to be effective (i.e., 40 mg/d or less).[9,27,42] Also, 10,794 clients were encouraged to detoxify from methadone 6 mo or less after their treatment began.

These results have several implications for policymakers and practitioners concerned with methadone maintenance treatment and the role of methadone treatment in HIV prevention. First, the results clearly indicate much variation in methadone treatment practices across the nation. These results, based on a nationally representative sample, are consistent with observations from studies that included limited samples of methadone units.[9,40] The key point is that many units have treatment practices that are not effective according to the majority of previous studies.[9,27,42,45] That is, many units have average dose levels and upper dose limits that are too low, and inflexible dose practices that are characterized by little input from clients. Second, our results are consistent with results from previous research that indicate the importance of dose level for client retention in treatment.[27,40,42,45] Units with higher average dose levels had longer average lengths of time in treatment for their clients. Length of time in treatment is critical: Results from several studies indicate that time in treatment is the strongest predictor of treatment success.

Third, characteristics of clients, treatment units, and their environments account for significant variation in treatment practices. Units that treat a higher percentage of young, male, and Black clients are less likely to have treatment practices that previous studies have found to be effective.

Results from several previous studies indicate that older clients remain in treatment longer,[46] and results from a recent study of 606 methadone maintenance clients from 21 clinics indicate that the rate of retention in treatment for Black clients was only 79% of the retention rate for non-Black clients.[47] D'Aunno and Vaughn's results may explain why young and Black clients are not remaining in treatment: They are more likely to receive restrictive treatment. Moreover, their results may explain why Blacks are more likely to be infected with the HIV virus.[48] That is, the results suggest that the type of methadone treatment Black clients are receiving may be contributing to their HIV infection rates by reducing their length of time in treatment.

Some unit characteristics are associated with a mixed pattern of treatment practices. On the one hand, free-standing units have lower dose limits and less client participation in setting dose levels; similarly, public units have lower average dose levels. On the other hand, however, both free-standing and public units have longer average time in treatment for their clients. Further study of free-standing and public units is needed to determine how they are able to retain clients in treatment despite somewhat restrictive treatment practices.

Units that are located in rural areas and in the South Atlantic and East North Central (i.e., Illinois, Indiana, Michigan, Ohio, and Wisconsin) states are also less likely to be effective. One interpretation for such regional variation is that program directors and staff members may belong to regional professional associations that foster a particular treatment philosophy. Similarly, geographic proximity may promote informal contact among staff members and managers, which shapes a regional treatment philosophy.

Finally, the role of government regulation is important. Units with higher dose limits and higher average dose levels are more likely to report that their dose practices are influenced by government regulation. In our view, the results of this study suggest that steps should be taken to monitor and, if necessary, change the treatment practices of methadone maintenance units that are providing inadequate dose levels with little client input. Further, this study identifies the types of units that are engaging in practices that put their clients at greater risk for failure in treatment.

There is an emerging consensus that methadone treatment is an important way to prevent HIV transmission. Preventing HIV transmission depends, however, on retaining clients in treatment. D'Aunno and Vaughn's results, as well as results from other studies, show that effective retention depends on adequate dose levels.

The Role of Drug Abuse Treatment Units in HIV Prevention

One of the most significant challenges that the drug abuse treatment faces is to respond to the AIDS epidemic. In particular, data from the Centers for Disease Control continue to indicate that iv drug users are a high-risk group for acquiring and transmitting HIV.[49] One key way to reach this high-risk group is through the nation's network of outpatient drug abuse treatment units.[36] These units treated an estimated 183,000 needle-users in 1989.[50] Further, through their clients, these units may have access to many of the approx 1 million needle-users who are not in treatment.

A recent survey of state offices of substance abuse treatment indicated that there are a variety of state and federal efforts to support the role of treatment units in HIV prevention.[50] The National Institute on Drug Abuse (NIDA), for example, has provided units with special training for staff members and funds to hire prevention specialists.[51] On the whole, however, we know very little about the responses of these units to the HIV epidemic. What prevention efforts are they engaged in? For example, are units providing HIV antibody testing and counseling for clients? Are they attempting to reach iv drug users who are not in treatment?

Given the central role that outpatient drug abuse treatment units can play in HIV prevention and our lack of understanding of their actual prevention efforts, the national study of outpatient drug abuse treatment units addressed two questions. First, to what extent are these treatment units engaged in various types of HIV prevention efforts? Second, what factors promote or inhibit HIV prevention efforts by these treatment units?

Data to address these questions were drawn from a national random sample of 575 treatment units that participated in a survey conducted in the Fall of 1988 by the University of Michigan's Institute for Social Research. Unit clinical supervisors completed phone surveys regarding their unit's HIV prevention practices; the survey response rate was 85.8%.

The data indicate that the majority of units (53%) routinely counsel clients on HIV prevention. In contrast, relatively few units (17%) have special staff members for HIV prevention efforts to provide HIV antibody testing. Of the units, 39% are involved in multiple efforts to reach drug users not in treatment, but results indicate that units devote relatively few hours per week (less than 10 on average) to such efforts, and only 78 units distribute bleach or condoms or try to reach iv drug users in such places as crack houses.

Results of regression analyses indicate that several factors—staff training, the availability of special staff and funds, client risk factors (especially iv drug use), and managerial support—account for significant variation in units' prevention practices. Implications of these findings include the following.

First, these results suggest that funds and programs devoted to staff training and education are having their desired impact on HIV prevention efforts. Drug abuse treatment units whose staff members have had special training or units with special staff are much more likely to engage in HIV prevention efforts both with their clients and with drug users not in treatment. These results indicate the importance of continuing state and federal efforts to hire HIV prevention specialists or drug abuse treatment units and to train staff members in treatment units for HIV prevention practices.

The results also suggest that units with clients at high risk for HIV infection (i.e., iv drug users, minorities) are more likely to engage in prevention efforts than units whose clients are not so much at risk. Though we anticipated this finding, it is, in our view, a "mixed blessing." On the one hand, it is critical for units to focus prevention efforts on high-risk groups; on the other hand, HIV prevention efforts with other drug users should not be neglected.

Further, after taking client characteristics into account, there is relatively little urban–rural and regional variation in HIV prevention efforts. That is, the results indicate that there are few significant differences among units' prevention efforts that can be attributed to geographic location, with two important exceptions: Urban units are likely to have a greater total number of outreach efforts and more collaborative efforts. Units located in more rural areas both have fewer clients at risk and are engaging in somewhat fewer prevention efforts than units located in more urban areas. Thus, our results have particular implications for policymakers and practitioners concerned with HIV prevention in rural areas. Prevention efforts in such areas may need to be increased.

Controversy continues, because many professionals in the drug abuse treatment field are opposed to any prevention efforts that they believe may increase drug use: Needle-exchange programs and the distribution of clcan nccdlcs and blcach solutions are frequently opposed on these grounds. Clinical supervisors in 30% of the units in our sample did not support the distribution of clean needles, bleach solutions, or condoms to iv drug users. Another 195 supervisors reported that they support such prevention efforts only "to some extent." Only about 35% of all clinical supervisors give unqualified support for these outreach efforts. Our results indicate that such beliefs are important predictors of variation in outreach practices. The implication is clear: The role of drug abuse treatment units in HIV prevention will continue to be limited if their leaders remain opposed to available prevention efforts because of their beliefs about possible encouragement of drug use.

There is a need for more fine-grained analysis of the processes involved in particular HIV prevention practices. For example, we know very little about HIV testing and counseling done in drug abuse treatment units. How well qualified and well trained are the counselors? Is testing mandatory or voluntary in units where testing is done at all? To what extent is confidentiality safeguarded?

Finally, most units are not extensively involved in such prevention efforts. This study indicates that interventions to increase the role of drug abuse treatment units in HIV prevention should take into account characteristics of units as well as their clients and staff members.

Ownership and Financing of Drug Abuse Treatment Services

Treatment Efficiency and Access

One of the major policy changes that has occurred in the 1980s has been the decision to rely much more heavily on the private sector for the delivery or management of traditionally public services.[52] Although much of the debate about this policy decision has gone on in the context of health services, the decision to rely on the private sector has covered a wide range of traditionally publicly supported services, including utilities, refuse collection, and housing. Much of the support for the privatization decision has been owing to beliefs about the advantages to be gained by private sector provision. Donahue[53] has reviewed these arguments, many of which revolve around the belief that more efficient services can be provided by private sector programs because of their susceptibility to market influences. Cost effectiveness, it can be argued, can come from a wide variety of aspects of the market, including increased economies of scale, purchasing, and development, as well as more efficient executive management and use of labor. Competition in the market in the private sector is believed to be superior to public or not-for-profit sectors because of increased pressure to control costs and prices.

Weisner and Room[54] and Ferris and Graddy[55] have observed that a substantial proportion of substance abuse treatment services are delivered by private providers, and the recent Institute of Medicine Report[1] has observed that the national system of drug abuse treatment has developed into a "two-tier" system of private and public supply. The private tier of drug treatment is oriented primarily, they argue, to treating the employed population and their family members.

On the other hand, Gerstein and Harwood[1] observed that public coverage is justified on two basic principles. First, public coverage should seek to reduce external costs of drug abuse, particularly those having to do with crime and role dysfunction in the family. Second, public coverage should allow persons with inadequate income to obtain treatment. Since there are approx 35 million individuals in the US who may qualify as indigent because they are neither adequately insured or able to pay out-of-pocket for appropriate forms of specialized drug abuse treatment, the justification for public coverage seems strong.

Despite the debates about the efficiency and effectiveness of publicly vs privately provided service, little is known about the drug abuse treatment sector when it comes to this critical distinction. However, the 1988 Drug Abuse Treatment System Survey included public sector outpatient treatment organizations; private not-for-profit organizations; and private for-profit drug treatment organizations in its sample. In addition, the survey collected extensive information about treatment costs and the financing of treatment. As a consequence, these survey data allow us to draw some conclusions about the nature of differences in public vs private treatment auspices, as well as information about revenue arrangements, efficiency of service delivery, and access. In addition, we can assess the effect of different payment systems and payment incentives on the organization of services.

Differences Between for-Profit and Not-for-Profit Units

Burke and Rafferty[56] contrasted public programs with private for-profit and private not-for-profit programs using the 1988 DATSS data. The most pervasive and persistent differences among units are those that distinguish for-profit units from both nonprofit and public units. Burke and Rafferty observe that the private sector is really two sectors, not one, and that for-profit status is the decisive variable distinguishing among public, private, not-for-profit, and private for-profit treatment units. Their analyses indicate that private for-profit units are more likely to rely on private sources of funding, including client fees and private insurance. Private for-profit units are also less likely to depend on referrals from the courts, police, and social service agencies. The DATSS data also suggest that for-profit units serve a distinctly different clientele than do nonprofit and public units. A smaller proportion of for-profit clients are under 20, are unemployed, are unable to pay for treatment, or have multiple drug problems. For-profit units serve a less disabled, less vulnerable pool of clients who have more financial resources.

Revenue Arrangements, Efficiency, Access to Care and Services Offered in Relationship to Ownership Status

Wheeler et al.[57] have conducted an additional study contrasting private for-profit units with public and not-for-profit units. Their results show that private for-profit units generate higher profits, charge higher prices, and may also operate at a higher efficiency level than public and private not-for-profit units. In contrast, public treatment units provide better access to care for persons who are unable to pay for care. It is also important to note that public and not-for-profit units appear to do more to facilitate access to care for people whose means of payment are limited by accepting a higher percentage of nonpayment and reduced fees.

In addition, Wheeler et al. found that private for-profit units provide a lower percentage of individual therapy sessions, which raises the question of whether this has any effect on the overall quality of care delivered. Fadel and Wheeler[58] found that pricing differences of the sort just described remain even after controlling for the effects of production, cost differences, differences in degree of competition for resources, differences in regulatory climate, and differences in patient characteristics. For-profit units charge substantially higher prices than private not-for-profit units, which, in turn, charge higher prices than public units.

Payment Systems, Payment Incentives, and Their Effects on Outpatient Substance Abuse Treatment

Another aspect of the organization of care that may affect the delivery of treatment is the nature of the payment system used in the reimbursement for treatment. Edlund et al.[59] examined the relationship between payment methods for treatment (for example, payment per treatment session) and the length of time clients are in treatment (for example, the average number of treatment sessions and their duration). Their results generally support the view that different payment methods provide varying incentives for treatment units to retain clients in treatment.

It is important to emphasize that retention in treatment is an important correlate of treatment effectiveness. Edlund et al. found treatment units with a higher percentage of revenue based on the number of clients and number of treatment visits are likely to provide more individual and group therapy sessions per client than units with higher percentages with revenue based on other payment methods. These results have important policy implications, because results from other studies[9] indicate that client time in treatment is the most important predictor of treatment effectiveness.

Conclusion

The recurring theme of this chapter is that the organization of drug abuse treatment services makes a substantial difference in who receives treatment, what services are provided, and how effective those services are. It appears that several organizational factors play important roles in shaping the provision of services. These factors include treatment unit ownership, location of units in various geographic and organizational settings (hospitals, mental health centers), staffing patterns, managerial beliefs, government regulation, and payment mechanisms.

It is also clear that we have just begun to understand what these organizational factors are and how they affect the delivery of drug abuse treatment services. Much of the organizational research reviewed herein, for example, does not consider inpatient or residential treatment units. Further, much of the research reviewed is cross-sectional and has not yet examined treatment units over time. Finally, the current organizational research on drug abuse treatment services does not focus enough on counselors or managers. More research is needed that is crosslevel, i.e., taking environmental, organizational, and staff characteristics into account. In short, there is a relatively large and important agenda for research on the organization of drug abuse treatment services.

Perhaps the most important item on this agenda should be to link organizational data to data from clients on treatment processes and outcomes. To date, the best studies of treatment effectiveness have not adequately taken into account organizational factors, such as unit ownership, location, and staffing patterns. That is, studies of treatment effectiveness fail to measure the impact of organizational factors on treatment processes or outcomes. On the other hand, studies of the organization of treatment services have not used individual-level client data to assess organizational effectiveness or efficiency. In our view, the time has certainly come to link organizational research to treatment research in a meaningful way. This would involve designing studies that have large representative samples of treatment units combined with large representative samples of clients receiving treatment in such units, and following both units and clients over time. Information from such studies could allow policymakers, managers, and clinicians to make more effective decisions concerning the organization and allocation of treatment resources (funds, staff), or, indeed, to lobby for more resources.

Acknowledgment

Preparation of this manuscript was supported by Grant R01 DA03272 from the National Institute on Drug Abuse.

References

[1]D. R. Gerstein and H. J. Harwood (eds.) (1990) *Treating Drug Problems: vol. 1. A Study of the Evolution, Effectiveness and Financing of Public and Private Drug Treatment Systems.* National Academy Press, Washington, DC.

[2]Drug Abuse Policy Office, Office of Policy Development, The White House (1984) *National Strategy for Prevention of Drug Abuse and Drug Trafficking.* US Government Printing Office, Washington, DC.

[3]F. M. Tims (1984) Introduction, in *Drug Abuse Treatment Evaluation: Strategies. Progress and Prospects* (NIDA Research Monograph 51). F. M. Tims and J. P. Ludford, eds. National Institute on Drug Abuse, Rockville, MD, pp. 9–12.

[4]T. A. D'Aunno and R. H. Price (1985) Organizational adaptation to changing environments: Community mental health and drug abuse services. *Am. Behav. Sci.* **28(5), May/June,** 669–683.

[5]J. H. Jaffee (1984) Evaluating drug abuse treatment: A comment on the state of the art, in *Drug Abuse Treatment Evaluation: Strategies. Progress and Prospects* (NIDA Research Monograph 51). F. M. Tims and J. P. Ludford, eds. National Institute on Drug Abuse, Rockville, MD.

[6]R. J. Frances (1988) Update on alcohol and drug disorder treatment. *J. Clin. Psychiatry* **49(9) Suppl.,** 13–17.

[7]R. H. Price, A. C. Burke, T. D'Aunno, D. M. Klingel, W. C. McCaughrin, J. A. Rafferty, and T. E. Vaughn (1989) *Outpatient Drug Abuse Treatment Services. 1988: Results of a National Survey* (NIDA Research Monograph 106). National Institute on Drug Abuse, Rockville, MD, pp. 63–92.

[8]M. Allison, R. L. Hubbard, and J. V. Rachal (1985) *Treatment Process in Methadone, Residential and Outpatient Drug Free Programs* (NIDA Research Monograph). National Institute on Drug Abuse, Rockville, MD.

[9]R. L. Hubbard, M. E. Marsden, J. V. Rachal, H. J. Harwood, E. R. Cavanaugh, and H. M. Ginzburg (1989) *Drug Abuse Treatment: A National Study of Effectiveness.* The University of North Carolina Press, Chapel Hill, NC.

[10]A. T. McLellan, L. Luborsky, G. E. Woody, and C. P. O'Brien (1980) An improved diagnostic evaluation instrument for substance abuse patients: The Addiction Severity Index. *J. Nerv. Ment. Disord.* **168,** 26–33.

[11]H. Ginzburg, M. Allison, and R. L. Hubbard (1984) Depressive symptoms in drug abuse treatment clinics: Correlates, treatment and changes, in *Problems of Drug Dependence: 1983* (NIDA Research Monograph 49). L. S. Harris, ed. National Institute on Drug Abuse, Rockville, MD, pp. 313–319.

[12]C. P. O'Brien, G. E. Woody, and A. T. McLellan (1984) *Psychotherapeutic approaches in the treatment of drug abuse* (NIDA Research Monograph 51). National Institute on Drug Abuse, Rockville, MD.

[13]G. E. Woody (1983) Treatment characteristics associated with outcome, in *Research on the Treatment of Narcotic Addiction.* J. R. Cooper, F. Altman, B. S. Brown, and D. Czechowicz, eds. U.S. Department of Health and Human Services, Rockville, MD, pp. 541–564.

[14]M. Allison, R. L. Hubbard, and S. G. Craddock, J. V. Rachal (1985) *Drug Abuse Treatment Process: Preliminary Examination of the TOPS Data* (RTI/1901/01–06S) Research Triangle Institute, Research Triangle Park, NC.

[15]G. W. Joe, D. D. Simpson, and S. B. Sells (in press) Treatment process and relapse to opioid use during methadone maintenance. *Am. J. Drug Alcohol Abuse.*

[16]M. K. Lehman (1990) Linking primary care and substance abuse treatment. *ADAMHA News* **16,** 1.

[17]J. Clement (1988) Corporate diversification: Expectations and outcomes. *Health Care Manage. Rev.* **13,** 7–13.

[18]B. Kissin, A. Platz, and W. H. Su (1970) Social and psychological factors in the treatment of chronic alcoholism. *J. Psychiatr. Res.* **8,** 13–27.

[19]H. M. Annis and D. Chan (1983) The differential treatment model: Empirical evidence from a personality typology of adult offenders. *Criminal Justice Behav.* **10,** 159–173.

[20]W. R. Miller, C. A. Taylor, and J. C. West (1980) Focused versus broadspectrum therapy for problem drinkers. *J. Consult. Clin. Psychol.* **48,** 590–601.

[21]R. K. Fuller, L. Branchey, D. R. Brightwell, R. M. Derman, C. D. Emrick, F. L. Iber, K. E. James, R. B. Lacoursiere, K. K. Lee, I. Lowenstam, I. Maany, D. Neiderhiser, J. J. Nocks, and S. Shaw (1986) Disulfiram treatment of alcoholism: A Veterans Administration cooperative study. *JAMA* **256,** 1449–1455.

[22]F. S. Gilbert (1988) The effect of type of aftercare follow-up on treatment outcome among alcoholics. *J. Stud. Alcohol* **49,** 149–159.

[23]W. R. Miller and R. K. Hester (1986) Inpatient alcoholism treatment: Who benefits? *Am. Psychol.* **41,** 794–805.

[24]W. C. McCaughrin and R. H. Price (1990) *Effective Outpatient Drug Abuse Treatment Organizations: Program Features and Selection Effects.* Drug Abuse Treatment System Survey working paper. University of Michigan, Survey Research Center, Institute for Social Research, Ann Arbor, MI.

[25]J. A. Liappas, F. A. Jenner, and B. Vicente (1988) Literature on methadone maintenance clinics. *Int. J. Addict.* **23,** 927–940.

[26]V. P. Dole, M. E. Nyswander, D. Des Jarlais, and H. Joseph (1982) Performance based rating of methadone maintenance programs. *N. Engl. J. Med.* **306,** 169–172.

[27]W. A. Hargreaves (1983) Methadone dose and duration for maintenance treatment, in *Research on the Treatment of Narcotic Addiction.* J. R. Cooper, F. Altman, B. S. Brown, and D. Czechowicz, eds. US Department of Health and Human Services, Rockville, MD, pp. 19–79.

[28]V. P. Dole (1988) Implications of methadone maintenance for theories of narcotic addiction. *JAMA* **260,** 3025–3029.
[29]R. G. Newman (1987) Methadone treatment: Defining and evaluating success. *N. Engl. J. Med.* **317,** 447–450.
[30]D. D'Amanda (1983) Program policies and procedures associated with treatment outcome, in *Research on the Treatment of Narcotic Addiction.* J. R. Cooper, F. Altman, B. S. Brown, and D. Czechowicz, eds. US Department of Health and Human Services, Rockville, MD, pp. 637–679.
[31]M. A. Rosenbaum (1985) A matter of style: Variation among methadone clinics in the control of clients. *Contemp. Drug Problems* **12,** 375–399.
[32]L. K. Altman (1989) U.S. to ease methadone rules in bid to curb AIDS in addicts. *The New York Times,* **March 3,** 1,9.
[33]A. S. Abdul-Quader, S. R. Friedman, D. C. Des Jarlais, M. M. Marmor, R. Maslansky, and S. Bartelme (1987) Methadone maintenance and behavior by intravenous drug users that can transmit HIV. *Contemp. Drug Problems* **14,** 425–434.
[34]S. Yancovitz, D. Des Jarlais, N. Peyser, P. Friedman, H. L. Trigg, and W. Robinson (1991) A randomized trial of an interim methadone maintenance clinic. *Am. J. Public Health* **81,** 1185–1191.
[35]S. L. Bakti, J. L. Sorensen, C. Coates, and D. Gibson (1988) *Methadone Maintenance for AIDS Affected IV Drug Users: Treatment Outcome and Psychiatric Factors after Three Months.* Paper presented at the 50th Annual Meeting of the Committee on the Problems of Drug Dependence, North Falmouth, MA, June.
[36]D. C. Des Jarlais, S. R. Friedman, and C. Casriel (1990) Target groups for preventing AIDS among intravenous drug users: 2. The "hard" data studies. *J. Consult. Clin. Psychol.* **58,** 50–56.
[37]C. R. Schuster (1988) Intravenous drug use and AIDS prevention. *Public Health Rep.* **103,** 261–266.
[38]D. C. Des Jarlais, H. Joseph, and V. P. Dole (1981) Long-term outcomes after termination from methadone maintenance treatment. *Ann. NY Acad. Sci.* **362,** 231–238.
[39]D. D. Simpson, J. L. Savage, and S. B. Sells (1978) *Data Book on Drug Treatment Outcomes: Follow-up Study of 1969–1972 Admissions to the Drug Abuse Reporting Program (DARP)* (Rep. No. 78–10) Texas Christian University, Institute of Behavior Research, Fort Worth, TX.
[40]J. C. Ball, W. R. Lange, C. P. Myers, and S. R. Friedman (1988) Reducing the risk of AIDS through methadone maintenance treatment. *J. Health Soc. Behav.* **29,** 214–226.
[41]J. K. Watters (1986) *Treatment Environment and Client Outcome in Methadone Maintenance Clinics.* Unpublished doctoral dissertation, University of Michigan.

[42]V. P. Dole (1989) Methadone treatment and the acquired immunodeficiency syndrome epidemic. *JAMA* **262,** 1681,1682.

[43]J. R. Cooper, F. Altman, B. S. Brown, and D. Czechowicz (eds.) (1983) *Research on the Treatment of Narcotic Addiction.* US Department of Health and Human Services, Rockville, MD.

[44]T. D'Aunno and T. E. Vaughn (1990) *Variation in Methadone Treatment Practices: Results from a National Study.* Drug Abuse Treatment System Survey working paper. University of Michigan, Survey Research Center, Institute for Social Research, Ann Arbor, MI.

[45]J. R. Cooper (1989) Methadone treatment and acquired immunodeficiency syndrome. *JAMA* **262,** 1664–1668.

[46]T. A. McLellan (1983) Patient characteristics associated with outcome, in *Research on the Treatment of Narcotic Addiction.* J. R. Cooper, F. Altman, B. S. Brown, and D. Czechowicz, eds. US Department of Health and Human Services, Rockville, MD, pp. 541–564.

[47]G. W. Joe, D. D. Simpson, and R. L. Hubbard (1990) *Treatment Predictors of Tenure in Methadone Maintenance.* Unpublished manuscript, Texas Christian University, Institute of Behavioral Research, Fort Worth, TX.

[48]E. E. Schoenbaum, D. Hartel, Selwyn, et al. (1989) Risk factors for human immunodeficiency virus infection in intravenous drug users. *N. Eng. J. Med.* **321,** 874–879.

[49]Centers for Disease Control. *Morbidity Mortality Weekly Rep.* **39,** 26.

[50]J. K. Watters, M. Reilly, and T. D'Aunno (1989) *AIDS Prevention Activities for Intravenous Drug Users in Treatment Programs: A National Survey of State Drug Abuse Administrators.* Center for AIDS Prevention Studies, University of California at San Francisco.

[51]J. Liebman, D. S. McIlvaine, L. Kotranski, and R. Lewis (1990) AIDS prevention for IV drug users and their sexual partners in Philadelphia. *Am. J. Public Health* **80,** 615–616.

[52]L. S. Simons (1989) Privatization and the mental health system. *Am. Psychol.* **44,** 1138–1141.

[53]J. D. Donahue (1989) *The Privatization Decision.* Basic, New York.

[54]C. Weisner and R. Room (1984) Financing and ideology in alcohol treatment. *Soc. Problems* **32,** 167–184.

[55]J. Ferris and E. Graddy (1986) Contracting out: For what? With whom? *Public Administration Rev.* **46,** 332–344.

[56]A. C. Burke and J. Rafferty (1990) *Ownership Differences in the Organization and Provision of Outpatient Substance Abuse Services.* University of Michigan, Survey Research Center, Institute for Social Research, Ann Arbor, MI.

[57]J. R. C. Wheeler, H. Fadel, and T. A. D'Aunno (1990) *Ownership and Performance in Outpatient Substance Abuse Centers.* Drug Abuse Treatment System Survey working paper. University of Michigan, Survey Research Center,

Institute for Social Research, Ann Arbor, MI.

[58]H. Fadel and J. R. C. Wheeler (1991) *Pricing Behavior of Outpatient Substance Abuse Treatment Organizations.* Drug Abuse Treatment System Survey working paper. University of Michigan, Survey Research Center, Institute for Social Research, Ann Arbor, MI.

[59]M. Edlund, J. R. C. Wheeler, and T. A. D'Aunno (1992) Payment systems and payment incentives in outpatient substance abuse treatment. *Public Budgeting Financial Manage* **4,** 107–123.

Development of an Information Strategy for the Drug Treatment System

James M. Kaple

Substance abuse treatment has become a principal part of the drug demand reduction strategy in the United States. At the same time, drug treatment is not well understood or openly embraced by the full range of public and private purchasers of health care services. Recent Institute of Medicine (IOM) analysis[1-3] of the nation's drug abuse treatment system and related research opportunities underlines the need for extensive services research and data development activities to better inform those responsible for financing and managing public and private access to health care.

Lessons learned in other health care delivery areas demonstrate the power and importance of services data and services research to inform and guide policy. Many of the widely accepted services and management reforms in the general health care delivery system today were promoted by data developed and services research conducted at the Health Care Financing Administration (HCFA) over the past 15 years. For example:

- Hospital payment reform options were developed and evaluated, and diagnosis-related groups (DRGs) were adopted.

From: *Drug and Alcohol Abuse Reviews, Vol. 4: Drug Abuse Treatment*
Ed: R. R. Watson ©1992 The Humana Press Inc.

- Coverage was expanded to include such new providers and services as ambulatory surgery centers, hospice care, and second-opinion programs.
- New quality assessment and outcome indicators for inpatient services, such as case-mix-adjusted death rates and nosocomial and iatrogenic complication rates, were developed and employed.

The information derived from treatment/services data and services research employing this data have proven useful in informing policy-making that affects change in the health care delivery system.

This chapter suggests some options for the development of an information strategy specifically for the drug treatment field. Three questions come to mind when one thinks about such an information strategy:

- Why are we interested in drug treatment/services information?
- What comprises a drug treatment/services information strategy?
- How should such an information strategy be developed and implemented?

Each of these questions is addressed in turn.

Why Drug Treatment/Services Information?

One might ask why policymakers are just now demanding improved information on the drug treatment/services system. Over the last decade, we have seen a significant increase in both the public and private investment in drug abuse treatment. On the private side, substance abuse treatment cost, as a share of total health care costs, escalated rapidly during the 1980s (in excess of 32% from 1986 to 1988).[4] In 1986, Krizay[5] estimated that substance abuse cost the insurance industry in excess of $50 billion a year. On the public side, nominal state and federal expenditures for drug abuse treatment have more than doubled in the last decade.[1]

Recently, the Public Health Service (PHS) initiated a series of task force meetings designed "to promote the availability of data in high priority public health policy areas over the next several years"[6] The very first "high priority" area chosen for review by the Public Health Service was that of drug abuse data. The report, which was released approximately 1 year ago, focused primarily on the drug-related data collection efforts within the Department of Health and Human Services. The Executive Summary states, "the core family of PHS drug abuse surveys, monitoring, and surveillance activities has met many basic data needs for a number of years." However, "increasing policy attention to drug abuse prevention and treatment has resulted in emerging data needs that are not being adequately addressed by current systems."

A subsequent expert-consensus report by the Rand Corporation, published in June 1990, titled, "Improving Data for Federal Drug Policy Decisions,"[7] reached a somewhat more critical conclusion. They stated:

> Policymakers have been handicapped by inconsistent and fragmented information on the extent and nature of drug problems and on programs aimed at controlling it. . . . Little is known about the effects different kinds of control programs (enforcement, treatment, and prevention) have on the drug problem. (p. 1)

At the same time, the two recent congressionally mandated IOM reports[1,3] suggest that Medicaid drug treatment coverage be expanded, and that private insurance carriers consider broadening the array of eligible drug treatment providers and the removal of discriminatory financial barriers, such as higher copays and deductibles. Many believe these changes will not be made on blind faith, but will require improved treatment/services information to respond to the tough questions raised by those charged with fiscal responsibility for these programs.

With rapidly escalating private and public costs has come increased demand for accountability and cost-effectiveness in the delivery of drug abuse treatment. In the private sector, such information is needed to guide insurance coverage, reimbursement, and treatment access decisions for commercial insurers and Blue Cross plans. In the public sector, this information is needed to inform public policy decisions involving program planning and the relative emphasis placed on different treatment strategies. Furthermore, even if these questions did not exist, the ongoing administrative, management, and billing requirements associated with expanded coverage include fundamental, comparable information on each client for whom services are delivered.

Finally, improved information would assist treatment system managers and clinicians in meeting their information needs, both for accountability purposes and in describing and managing their treatment caseloads. If carefully designed and implemented, these various needs for treatment data can be addressed simultaneously.

Thus, the answer to the "why" question is: Policymakers and experts reviewing drug treatment/services issues are demanding more and improved information as they consider national priorities *vis-à-vis* drug abuse supply and demand reduction strategies, and as they respond to demands for expanded drug treatment coverage, such as that called for in the IOM reports (i.e., expanded eligibility, coverage, and reimbursement).

What Comprises a Drug Treatment/Services Information Strategy?

Treatment/services data requirements include information on clients in treatment, the treatment process, costs, and the structure of the treatment system. Data on epidemiological population trends in drug use behavior do not fulfill this requirement. Clinical trials data do not fulfill this requirement. Although there should be careful coordination of treatment information with that of epidemiology, clinical research, criminal justice, prevention, and potentially other informative areas, even the aggregate of these information elements cannot fulfill the requirement.

A reasonable and highly appropriate model for meeting the requirement exists in the general medical care sector. When the Medicare and Medicaid programs were initiated in the mid-1960s, the federal government and every citizen acquired an increasing stake in the medical care delivery system. Many questions similar to those now raised about drug abuse treatment were asked: What services should be covered? What providers should be eligible to deliver care? How should it be paid for? How much should be paid? How could the system be improved over time? To answer these questions significant investments have been and continue to be made in data development and health services research. The results are striking both for the policy changes they brought about, and the impact they have had on the data and information collection systems in the general medical care sector. It is from the perspective of health services research that a long-range information strategy for the drug treatment field can be most efficiently developed and implemented.

The kinds of changes mentioned earlier (first in the federal Medicare program, and later in Blue Cross and commercial insurance)—that is, decisions to cover and pay for ambulatory surgery; adoption of second-opinion surgery programs; expansion of coverage to hospice care; the movement to DRG-based payment mechanisms for in-hospital services; and most recently, the focus on outcome measurement, quality, and appropriate patterns of health care delivery—grew in large part from the analysis of services and treatment data. Also, each of these changes brought with it its own specific impact on treatment data collection and analysis.

There is a symbiotic relationship among policy needs, services research, and data collection. This relationship has been clearly present in general medicine, and it is likely to be repeated in the drug treatment field. The function of health services research is to support and inform policy decisions. Health services research is data-dependent. The data needs and data acquisition strategies used in health services research often preview long-range, ongoing operational data requirements. We are just beginning to see the development of these requirements in the drug abuse field.

Three basic types of treatment/services data have been the mainstay of general medical care services research and are likely to become the focus for information needs in the drug treatment field. These three types of data are:

1. Client data;
2. Provider data; and
3. Outcome data.

Over time, data systems have developed and evolved in general medicine for each type of data. Client and provider data come directly from the treatment/services system. Outcome data are usually derived from special studies or longitudinal assessment of client and provider treatment data.

In the general medical system, at the client level, diagnostic and procedural data are recorded on hospital discharge forms and on physician and ambulatory billing forms. These discharge-based longitudinal data contain specified demographic information and are usually linkable to more detailed eligibility files. In the general medical care area, Medicare and Medicaid provider data systems were developed long ago to document the number and type of providers, the range of services, and the cost or charges for care delivered by these providers. Most recently, outcome data have been extended beyond the simple reporting of hospital discharge status to more sophisticated, multidimensional, case-mix-adjusted outcome variables.

The experience in the general medical care treatment community with client, provider, and outcome data could provide a framework for the development of a long-term information strategy for the drug treatment field. At the client level, individual client-discharge data could be standardized at the source, i.e., at the provider level. Expanded effort could be put into the development of a standard drug or alcohol client record. This could include client-specific information on the clinical characteristics of the patient (including diagnosis, drug history, and comorbid conditions), source of payment, measures of the quantity and type of services provider, and some quantification of the intensity and type of care administered.

Individual client-level data, to be most useful to support research and informed policymaking, must be collected at the time of discharge (and at established predischarge intervals when a long-term treatment is involved). To date, drug treatment provider capacity to maintain and provide such information in a uniform manner ranges widely.[8]

Care will be needed to reach consensus on the precise definition, content, and coding conventions to be used in such a client record. Training will be necessary to ensure that provider-based capacity exists to record and code accurate diagnostic, utilization, comorbidity, clinical, and charge-related data. Through standardization of client-level recordkeeping and documentation, and with the development of attendant Management Information System software, systems could be put in place to collect, manage, and make good use of this information at the facility level. This information could readily be transmitted to central data collection sources at local, state, and federal levels for management, health services research, and policy analytic purposes.

Such client-based information systems require safeguards for the protection of confidentiality (privacy). It should be noted that confidentiality issues have long been present in the general medical system and have been adequately dealt with to the point that they are no longer regarded as road blocks to the collection of necessary client-level information. Although the criminal dimensions of drug-related behavior create additional elements of concern about drug treatment records, there is an encouraging history of developing and maintaining confidential central records of drug client data.

With respect to provider-level data, revenue by source should be available, as well as information regarding the actual cost, charges, and range of services provided. Provider-level structural and process data, including staffing and credentialing information, should also be available. The capacity of facilities to capture such information and provide it to state, local, and federal policymakers and health services researchers varies widely. An important strategic step in improving the availability of provider data is the development of appropriate cost-finding and cost-allocation statistics, unit-of-service definitions, and data-collection methods.

It is critically important to develop operational definitions of treatment, service elements, and associated statistical units of measurement that adequately reflect the different approaches to treatment. Today's treatment definitions, which confuse phases of treatment, theoretical and philosophical orientations, particular pharmacological strategy, and site of treatment (e.g., outpatient drug-free, or residential), are inadequate to meet the policy and research needs of the treatment field. The methods for collecting, aggregating, and using such provider data should be approached in a systematic fashion similar to that adopted by the Medicare program as it established its provider of service and hospital cost-reporting information systems.

Outcome data pose unique challenges in the drug abuse field. Unlike general hospital medical care, very few drug abuse clients fail to survive drug treatment, and therefore, outcome measurements—such as "dead" or "alive" at date of discharge—have relatively little utility. Recent advances in measuring perceived quality-of-life, reliable urinalysis techniques, and the linkage with longitudinal data or postintervention consumption of other health resources, offer excellent tools for outcome assessment in the drug treatment field. Aside from the process and structure measures associated with treatment, it is understood that outcome data collection is outside the domain of the treatment systems, and will of necessity be captured by special studies or surveys—not by providers.

How Should a Strategy Be Developed?

Drug treatment/services information systems are necessary in supporting informed public and private policy decisions regarding access to, and reimbursement and coverage for, drug treatment. However, the development of ongoing data collection along the lines discussed earlier, if regarded solely as supporting research and informing policy decisions, is not realistic. To be viable, such data collection must occur as a byproduct of data systems that are integral to the provider's basic clinical, financial, and management records systems. We must develop the infrastructure to support efficient capture of high-quality, timely client and provider data at the source. This is precisely how successful provider and client-oriented data systems have evolved in the general medical field.

The treatment system in fact already collects and uses much of the necessary client and provider data; what needs to be done largely involves making these data more consistent, accurate, and retrievable. If such standardized data sets were developed, with input from the treatment providers, researchers, and the clinical community, they could serve the needs of both policy-level researchers and decisionmakers as well as the day-to-day management requirements at the clinical, case, and provider levels. In fact, the development of uniform systems of this type will enhance the ability of clinicians and treatment providers to understand and compare their own internal treatment decisions with those of their peers on both a regional and national level.

Such changes will require consensus building, since cooperation from the full range of provider, purchasing, and interest groups is required. One approach could involve the use of state or substate "laboratories," where a data-gathering infrastructure would be developed, tested, and evaluated. Such laboratories could provide a vehicle for local area collaboration, where diverse groups of providers, purchasers of care, researchers, and policymakers could assess alternative data-gathering methods. Results could be compared across sites, strengths and weaknesses assessed, and conclusions drawn about appropriate methods for broader implementation.

Summary

With care and commitment from policymakers, researchers, and providers, drug treatment/services data systems can be created that are compatible with the routine administrative, financing, and client data systems that serve ongoing management and clinical needs in the drug abuse field. Minimum data sets need to be established, and data quality and reliability measures should be built into the information collection process and the attendant management information systems. Although the focus of this discussion is client- and provider-level data, any drug abuse data strategy should be developed with an eye to the utility and ability to link with other data bases, including special survey outcome data, and basic biomedical and epidemiological data systems. Information may also be linked to such sources as state licensure, certification, and contract management systems. It is recognized that short-term and long-term surveys and special studies will continue to be necessary and appropriate to augment information collection that becomes a routine part of the drug treatment/services system.

A number of sources, including the two recently completed IOM reports,[1,2] urge that alcohol and drug treatment programs enter the mainstream of health care financing. Just as mainstream health care (whether publicly or privately financed) has complied with reasonable and necessary data requirements, part of the price for mainstream financing of drug treatment is likely to be high-quality, timely, comparable data on drug abuse clients, providers, and outcomes.

References

[1]D. R. Gerstein and J. Harwood (eds.) (1990) *Treating Drug Problems I: A Study of the Evolution, Effectiveness, and Financing of Public and Private Drug Treatment Systems.* Institute of Medicine, National Academy Press, Washington, DC.

[2]Institute of Medicine (US) (1989) *Prevention and Treatment of Alcohol Problems: Research Opportunities.* National Academy Press, Washington, DC.

[3]Institute of Medicine (US) (1990) *Broadening the Base of Treatment for Alcohol Problems.* National Academy Press, Washington, DC.

[4]R. Frank and D. Salkever (1991) Report on Expenditure and Utilization Patterns for Mental Illness and Substance Abuse Services under Private Health Insurance. American Psychiatric Association, Washington, DC

[5]Krizay, J. (1986) *The $50 Billion Drain: Alcohol. Drugs and the High Cost of Insurance.* Care Institute, CompCare Publications, Minneapolis, MN.

[6]US Public Health Service (1990) *Improving Drug Abuse Statistics.* Report of the PHS Task Force on Drug Abuse Data, February.

[7]J. Haaga and P. Reuter eds. (1991) *Improving Data for Federal Drug Policy Decisions.* RAND N-3241-BJS, RAND Drug Policy Research Center, Washington, DC.

[8]H. L. Batten, C. M. Horgan, and J. M. Prottas (1990) *Drug Services Research Survey Provisional Report: Phase I.* Bigel Institute for Health Policy, Brandeis University, under contract to National Institute on Drug Abuse, November 16.

Substance Abuse Relapse

Theory and Clinical Application

Jalie A. Tucker and Rudy E. Vuchinich

Introduction

Studies of substance abuse treatment effectiveness support the following generalizations[1–5]:

1. During the first several months after treatment, most clients show reduced substance use and improvements in related life problems.
2. By the end of the first year of posttreatment, however, up to 75% of clients have engaged in some substance use, with a substantial proportion having returned to pretreatment levels of abuse.
3. Outcome assessments at different follow-up points typically yield subgroups of clients who have maintained abstinence or who have engaged in variable substance use ranging from nonproblem to problem use. Over time, individual clients often move from one outcome category to another.
4. The type of outcome achieved does not vary substantially with the type of treatment received (e.g., 12-Step or behavioral), the intensity of treatment (e.g., inpatient or outpatient), or the stated goals of treatment (e.g., abstinence or moderation drinking goals).
5. Instead, treatment outcomes have a stronger relationship with client resources and environmental circumstances during the posttreatment period than with treatment-specific or client-intake characteristics.

From: *Drug and Alcohol Abuse Reviews, Vol. 4: Drug Abuse Treatment*
Ed: R. R. Watson ©1992 The Humana Press Inc.

These findings have forced a fundamental reorientation in clinical research on substance abuse disorders. Traditionally, relapse after treatment was attributed to extinction of treatment effects or to a failure of treatment-initiated changes to generalize to clients' natural environments.[6] If this were accurate, then "more, better, and longer-lasting applications of the original intervention"[6] (p. 9) should enhance the proportion of successful outcomes. This has not proven to be the case, and it now seems apparent that further modifications in existing treatments are not likely to improve long-term outcomes substantially, because the determinants of initial behavior change differ from those influencing long-term relapse and recovery patterns.[6] As a result, emphasis has shifted away from end point evaluations of treatment effectiveness toward research aimed at understanding how participation in time-limited treatments interacts with individuals' ongoing life circumstances, their motivations for behavior change, and the natural course of substance abuse over time.[7]

This revised view has focused attention on the discovery of variables that influence substance use patterns during the posttreatment interval and on devising strategies to eliminate or minimize substance use in clients' natural environments. Thus, research on the determinants of relapse has been at the core of this reorientation. This chapter describes the phenomena that need to be accounted for by models of the relapse process, summarizes historical accounts of relapse, and discusses four contemporary models. Then, contemporary clinical applications are described, along with the supporting evidence.

Models of the Relapse Process

Phenomena that Relapse Models Must Address

At a minimum, an adequate model of relapse should address three basic aspects of the process of resuming substance use after a period of abstinence. First, variables are required to explain why some former substance abusers reinitiate use and others do not. Second, among those who resume substance use, variables are required to explain the extent or severity of substance use episodes. Because some episodes end quickly without adverse consequences, whereas others entail a return to pretreatment patterns of abuse, a basis for distinguishing lapses from relapses[8] is essential, and variables that influence initial and continued consumption may differ in important ways. Third, relapse involves the resumption of substance use among individuals with an established problem history, and an account is required of how individuals' drug-taking histories may relate to their current substance use. Thus, models of relapse are likely to differ from accounts of the initial acquisition of substance abuse problems, although some common influences would certainly be expected.

In the discussion that follows, each model of relapse is described in the context of these basic requirements, and the empirical evidence bearing on each model is summarized. Because of the incipient stage of research on the relapse process, this presentation is not aimed at providing critical tests of one model over another. As we hope will be clear, the different models emphasize different aspects of the relapse process, often at different levels of analysis. The discussion highlights aspects of the relapse process that are best addressed by each model and notes their common and unique characteristics.

Historical Approaches to the Relapse Process

Nineteenth-century views of the "addict-as-fiend" contained assumptions about the relapse process that have survived in some contemporary literature, including the following:

1. An addict who lacked drug access would experience powerful drug cravings and would engage in escalating levels of drug-seeking behavior, regardless of the personal, economic, or other costs involved.
2. Once drug availability was secured, the addict would consume the drugs continuously without regard to other obligations.
3. When drug availability was once again constrained, declining drug effects or withdrawal symptoms would strongly motivate drug-seeking behavior, thus perpetuating the addiction cycle.

The disease model of alcoholism (summarized in ref. 9) incorporated many of these themes about the nature of addiction, and the view has been widely generalized to other substance abuse disorders. The disease model has an account of relapse that proposes separate mechanisms for the initiation of alcohol consumption after abstinence and for continued consumption to the point of intoxication. Abstinent alcoholics are held to experience repeated cravings for alcohol that eventually promote initial use. Initial use, in turn, precipitates loss of control over drinking that results in an inevitable return to abusive consumption. The disease model also fulfills the third criterion described earlier by positing a stable biological basis for this predisposition to drink uncontrollably, which is held to necessitate lifelong abstinence for recovering alcoholics.

Three separate lines of research during the 1960s and 1970s directly challenged the craving/loss-of-control model of relapse. First, Mello and Mendelson's (e.g., ref. 10) experimental studies of the drinking patterns of alcoholics showed that their alcohol consumption was influenced by its consequences and by other environmental contingencies. In contrast to the addict-as-fiend perspective, providing subjects with relatively minor incentives to restrict consumption reliably did so. Second, Marlatt et al.[11] demonstrated that alcoholics' beliefs of having consumed an initial dose of alcohol influenced their subsequent volitional alcohol consumption and that the actual ethanol content of the beverages did not affect consumption. This study directly questioned the loss-of-control notion that initial exposure to alcohol would physiologically trigger excessive drinking among alcoholics. Third, in 1962, Davies[12] reported that some treated gamma (i.e., physically dependent) alcoholics had maintained moderation-drinking outcomes. Subsequent treatment outcome studies have frequently observed moderation drinking outcomes for some subjects,[2,4,13] and occasional drug use without adverse consequences also has been noted with other substance abuse disorders.[14,15] These findings further questioned the disease model view that a biological predisposition compels lifelong abstinence for all substance abusers, although this goal is appropriate for many clients.

In addition to these empirical challenges, the craving/loss-of-control model of relapse has been criticized conceptually[16] as being descriptive at best and as being tautological if viewed as a causal explanation of the relapse process. Because of these limitations, the craving/loss-of-control account has fallen into disfavor in the psychological scientific literature, although it continues to dominate lay accounts.

Contemporary Theories of the Relapse Process

Dependence Syndrome Models

The alcohol dependence syndrome proposed by Edwards and colleagues[17,18] recently has been applied to the relapse process.[19,20] According to Edwards[17] (pp. 142–144), alcohol dependence lies on a continuum of severity involving seven elements that encompass biological, psychological, and behavioral variables. As dependence increases:

1. Drinking practices become more rigid and stereotypical (the drinking repertoire "narrows").
2. Drink-seeking behavior comes to dominate other behaviors.
3. Tolerance increases.
4. Withdrawal symptoms are experienced repeatedly.
5. "Relief drinking" occurs to avoid withdrawal symptoms.
6. Subjective awareness of the "compulsion" to drink increases.
7. When drinking beyond a "certain threshold of frequency and quantity" is initiated following abstinence, dependence symptoms reemerge with greater rapidity.

The dependence syndrome has implications for the relapse process, primarily as a result of hypothesis 7.[19,20] If individuals with high pretreatment dependence levels rapidly reestablish dependence symptoms when they resume substance use, then such persons should be poor candidates for moderation drinking and thus should be disportionately represented in outcome categories of sustained abstinence or relapse to abusive substance use.[20] Moreover, the speed with which dependence symptoms reemerge once substance use is resumed should be positively related to pretreatment levels of dependence,[19] and higher dependence levels should increase individuals' susceptibility to the effects of drug cues, including cues resulting from initial drug ingestion.[21,22]

As described later in the section on clinical applications, the central prediction concerning the relationship of dependence levels to moderation drinking outcomes after treatment has not received much empirical support,[13] although some limited support has been obtained for other predictions of the model. For example, the predicted association between pretreatment dependence levels and the speed and severity of dependence reinstatement once drinking is resumed has been found for male alcoholics, but not for opiate addicts or female alcoholics.[19] More consistent support has been observed for the prediction that higher dependence levels will increase alcoholics' susceptibility to alcohol cues. Rankin et al.[21] for example, found that severely dependent alcoholics consumed five drinks much faster than moderately dependent alcoholics. The investigators noted, however, that the rapid drinking of highly dependent alcoholics may have preceded and contributed to their development of dependence symptoms, which questions the value of the dependence syndrome as a controlling variable.

Another shortcoming of this account of relapse is that the conditions under which a previously abstinent alcoholic will reinitiate drinking are not specified. Babor et al.[19] attempted to resolve this shortcoming by incorporating key concepts of other relapse models (i.e., efficacy expectations, conditioned withdrawal effects), but these notions lack conceptual coherence with the dependence model, are *ad hoc*, and, in the case of conditioned withdrawal effects, have not been supported as influential in the relapse process *(see* Motivational–Conditioning Models section later in this chapter). Importantly, because the dependence model lacks explicit criteria for determining the conditions under which initial substance use is more likely, the utility of the concept for developing relapse prevention strategies is limited.

Finally, the dependence syndrome has been criticized on numerous other grounds,[13,23–26] including:

1. Despite disclaimers to the contrary, it is conceptually similar to the disease model of alcoholism in proposing a stable, largely biological predisposition for substance abuse and thus diminishes necessary emphasis on psychosocial and environmental factors known to influence substance disorders.
2. Like the craving/loss-of-control model of relapse, the dependence syndrome is circular in that abusive drinking is viewed as evidence of dependence, which then is used to explain abusive drinking.
3. Only the more biological elements of the syndrome have been supported empirically.

Overall, empirical support for applications of the dependence syndrome to relapse must be considered very limited.

Stress–Coping Models

Stress–coping models of relapse[16,27–29] generally adopt the assumptions of Lazarus'[30] classic work on stress and coping and regard substance use as one response that may be emitted to cope with perceived threat. Although the different versions of the approach vary in terms of the mechanisms thought to promote relapse, their common focus is on the interaction over time between relapse-risk factors and relapse-protective factors. Depending on the specific model, relapse-risk factors may include perceived stress levels and negative affect, high-risk situations associated with past substance use or with current cues for substance use, lack of coping responses other than substance use to deal with high-risk situations or perceived stress, positive expectations of the effects of substance use, and low self-efficacy for avoiding substance use. Relapse-protective factors generally focus on alternative cognitive and behavioral coping responses that may be emitted in the immediate high-risk situation for substance use. Thus, when an individual encounters a high-risk situation, the probability of substance use will vary with the perceived degree of threat or stress, the availability of alternative coping responses, and the individual's expectations about the relative effectiveness of substance use vs alternative responses to cope with the perceived threat.

Once substance use occurs, the different versions of the approach provide a basis for distinguishing relapse severity. According to Marlatt's[16,28] well known model of relapse, whether an initial lapse develops into a protracted relapse will depend on the outcome of a complex sequence of cognitive and affective reactions to the initial use known as the *abstinence violation effect*; the stronger the violation effect, the greater the probability of an extended relapse. In Annis and Davis'[27] model, the probability and severity of relapse are held to vary with clients' self-efficacy expectations for avoiding substance use in specific situations associated with past substance use. Ratings of self-efficacy obtained at or shortly after treatment termination have been found to predict the situations in which posttreatment relapses occur.[31,32] Finally, Shiffman[29] characterized individuals' "relapse proneness" over time as a function of a complex interplay between stable individual characteristics (e.g., problem severity), changeable background factors (e.g., stress levels), and transitory precipitating events (e.g., substance cues). Whether or not substance use will occur and the severity of the episode will depend on the interaction of these variable classes at any point in time.

A core feature of all stress–coping models is an emphasis on individuals' cognitive and affective reactions and coping responses in the immediate high-risk situation for substance use. Although these temporally contiguous responses in high-risk situations may be influenced by historical forces or by variables that operate over longer time frames, stress–coping models focus on individuals' cognitive–affective state during substance availability as the critical determinant of relapse. Such a focus is consistent with the many studies that have observed positive relationships between relapse episodes and stressful events, negative affective states, and other characteristics of the immediate substance use situation.[33,34] However, as discussed next, these same data are subject to at least two alternative explanations and cannot be viewed as exclusive support for stress–coping models.

Motivational–Conditioning Models

Motivational-conditioning models of relapse[35–38] hypothesize that the activation of motivational states by certain environmental, biological, and/or affective stimuli initiates and maintains substance use. A basic assumption is that the motivational state is conditionable to stimuli associated with substance use episodes and that such stimuli will come to elicit the motivational state that directs behavior toward substance use. If, after treatment, an individual encounters stimuli paired with past substance use, the motivational state presumably will be activated and will lead to resumed use, the severity of which will depend on properties of the state. Activation of the state with high intensity and long duration will facilitate an extended relapse, whereas activation with low intensity and short duration will result in more limited drug use.

The versions of the approach differ in the mechanisms proposed to underlie the relapse process. Early accounts[36] posited that the primary motivation is to escape from or to avoid withdrawal symptoms. Thus, when stimuli associated with past drug withdrawal are encountered, the probability of relapse should increase. However, because the predicted relationship between relapse and environmental cues associated with withdrawal symptoms has not been well supported, more recent models have proposed that the primary motivation is to experience the positive effects of substances.[35,37,38] When stimuli associated with the past experience of positive substance effects are encountered, the probability of relapse should increase. Research to date better supports the latter, incentive motivation view over a withdrawal avoidance interpretation.[37,38]

Certain motivational models also assign a key role to affective states in the relapse process.[35] To the extent that positive and negative affect are similar to the motivational states associated with drug withdrawal and with positive substance effects, respectively, the affective states may motivate substance use, either because they mimic the motivational state or because they serve as conditioned stimuli for its elicitation. The environmental conditions that produce the affective states presumably do not have to be those associated with past substance use or withdrawal. Therefore, any environmental context that produces relevant affective changes is predicted to increase the probability of relapse, in addition to the influence of stimuli directly associated with past drug withdrawal or positive substance effects. As such, like the stress–coping models, motivational models provide an account of the frequently observed relationship between relapse and negative affective states and stressful events, although the proposed mechanism is different. In addition, motivational models provide an interpretation of the association observed between a smaller percentage of relapse episodes and positive affective states.[16]

Behavioral Choice Model

Behavioral theories of choice[39] seek to explain how the behavior of individuals is allocated among a set of available alternatives that vary in the constraints on their access. A key assumption that is firmly supported by research[40] is that behavioral allocation to any given alternative is context-dependent. Allocation to a given activity will depend on what other activities are available and on the relative constraints associated with engaging in each alternative. As applied to substance abuse and relapse,[41] the basic issue is to identify the environmental conditions under which substance use emerges as the preferred activity from among the available set. Research on drug self-administration with human and animal subjects has revealed two general relationships between drug preference and the surrounding environmental conditions[41]: Drug preference varies directly with substance accessibility and inversely with the accessibility of alternative reinforcers. Conditions that promote a strong preference for substance use thus should entail minimal direct constraints on substance availability and few alternative reinforcers and/or increased constraints on access to them.

This view suggests that the probability of relapse after treatment should increase (1) when individuals enter situations in which the substance is immediately available at low cost and (2) when events occur that indicate increased constraints on access to valued alternative activities, especially those activities whose receipt is dependent in part on continued abstinence or nonproblem substance use. The model also predicts that the two types of environmental conditions should result in substance use episodes of different severity. Substance use episodes associated only with immediate substance availability should be less severe than those also associated with increased constraints on access to alternative reinforcers. In the former situation, there has been no overall change in access to valued alternative rewards; once an individual leaves the situation with immediate substance cues, preference should revert back to behaving in ways (e.g., maintaining abstinence) that increase the likelihood of receipt of valued alternatives. In the latter case, however, access to the alternative rewards has become constrained, and preference for substance use should remain higher over a longer time period. This differential prediction concerning the circumstances associated with substance use episodes of varying severity has been supported in studies of the determinants of alcohol[42] and smoking[43] relapse.

Discussion of the Models

Conceptual Adequacy

These four models of relapse include hypothesized influences on the severity of relapse episodes once drug use has been resumed and an account of how individuals' substance abuse histories may be related to current use. Only the dependence syndrome model fails to include an explicit account of variables that influence the initiation of drug use after a period of abstinence.

With respect to the determinants of relapse severity, the dependence syndrome model appeals to individuals' pretreatment levels of dependence as a controlling variable, but, as noted earlier, the logic of this assumption appears circular and thus at best descriptive. The stress–coping and motivational models posit somewhat different mechanisms, but share a common focus on temporally contiguous influences that operate in the immediate drug use situation. The behavioral choice perspective, in contrast, addresses the lapse–relapse distinction by differentiating factors that lie in the environmental conditions that exist before and when substance use begins. By offering a basis for predicting relapse severity prior to the onset of substance use, the choice approach has potential advantages for relapse prevention.

With respect to individual substance use histories, the dependence model views past manifestations of the dependence syndrome as the critical influence on current drug use. An important and contentious issue in this literature[44] concerns whether dependence levels should be conceptualized as a stable trait or as a state variable that fluctuates over time. If viewed as a trait, then the dependence syndrome is subject to many of the same criticisms directed at disease-based explanations of substance abuse. If considered a state variable, then further specification of the variables that influence changing levels of dependence over time is clearly needed.

The remaining three models are more explicit about historical influences on current substance abuse patterns. Stress–coping models emphasize how specific situations associated with past substance use relate to positive expectations of substance effects and to present levels of self-efficacy to avoid drug use. Motivational models focus on environmental cues associated in the past with substance withdrawal or positive substance effects that serve to elicit current motivational states that direct behavior toward substance use. The behavioral choice model focuses on the contingencies that have been established in the past between substance abuse vs abstinence and the receipt of rewards in important areas of functioning. Although the current literature contains little evidence relevant to these various accounts, each model yields predictions that are amenable to empirical evaluation.

Regarding the controlling variables of initial substance use after treatment, the three models that directly address this issue share a common focus on environmental influences, but they differ in their interpretation of how environmental variables exert their effects. As discussed in the next section, a key difference concerns the extent to which environmental variables are viewed as having direct effects on behavior (behavioral choice perspective) or as being mediated through some internal state of the substance abuser in the drug-taking environment (stress–coping and motivational models). This issue notwithstanding, all three models share a common goal of explaining how posttreatment substance use patterns vary with the surrounding environment, an issue that is conspicuously absent in the dependence syndrome approach.

The Role of Affective States

A number of studies have reported positive correlations between relapse and negative affect or stressful events.[33,34] However, when the relationship of affective changes or negative events is studied in relation to discrete posttreatment substance use episodes,[42,45] it is clear that not all negative affective states or stressful events produce substance use, and, conversely, that not all substance use episodes are preceded or accompanied by such changes. Moreover, a limited proportion of substance use episodes are associated with positive, rather than negative, affect or events.[16]

Such data argue against a straightforward role for affect in the relapse process and necessitate a means of differentiating the conditions under which events and affective changes will and will not be associated with substance use. To address this issue, the stress–coping models rely on a basic explanatory device of Lazarus'[30] theory; i.e., environmental events will promote relapse only to the extent that they are *perceived* as a threat by the individual, and their effects will be further modified by the availability of alternative coping responses. Although the influence of alternative coping responses has received some support,[46,47] a curious finding in both event–relapse and general life stress research is that having subjects rate the perceived threat of events does not significantly increase the power of predicting relevant outcome variables.[48] Such findings question the role of this proposed perceptual process in mediating event–relapse relationships.

Motivational–conditioning models are similar to the stress–coping models in interpreting the relationship between stressful events and relapse as due to the effects of the events on internal states. Events or their associated affect may elicit the motivational state that promotes relapse, or increased levels of stress may lower the threshold required to activate the motivational state by environmental cues associated with past substance use or withdrawal. However, criteria for distinguishing when affective states will and will not elicit the motivational state that drives substance use are not specified. Without such criteria, the model has difficulty explaining why negative affect or stressful events fail to produce relapse in all instances.

The behavioral choice perspective adopts a much different strategy for addressing the role of affect and events in the relapse process. Whereas the stress–coping and motivational models view affective changes as a controlling variable in the relapse process, the choice perspective maintains that affective states may only be correlated with substance use episodes. Instead of focusing on the affective consequences of events, the choice model argues that the important dimensional properties of events with respect to relapse are what the events signal about changing constraints on individuals' future access to valued alternative activities. If a negative and stressful event has little consequence for individuals' access to valued alternatives, the probability of substance use should not change, whereas events signaling increased constraints on the alternatives should increase the likelihood of relapse. This view has received some preliminary support in a study of relapse determinants among alcoholics following inpatient treatment.[42]

More generally, compared to other relapse models, the choice perspective adopts a more molar view of the temporal dynamics of the relapse process. The other three models share a common emphasis on factors that operate either in the immediate high-risk situation for relapse or once substance use has begun. The choice model thus is probably best regarded as involving a different level of analysis than the other three models. It remains to be determined what relationships may exist between the more molar set of influences posited by the choice perspective and the more temporally contiguous set of variables hypothesized by the other models.

Relapse Protective Factors

Although the focus of relapse models is on the conditions that promote a return to substance use, variables that facilitate successful outcomes obviously are no less important. The treatment outcome literature has consistently found an association between maintenance of abstinence or nonproblem substance use and aspects of clients' posttreatment environmental circumstances and personal resources, including higher levels of vocational functioning, social stability, and family and marital functioning.[4,49,50] Also, reduced substance use often is associated with decreases in other life problems,[51,52] although the correlational nature of these data precludes determination of causal relationships.

Specifying the conditions that facilitate recovery would appear to be a fundamental requirement of relapse models, but this issue has only been addressed explicitly by the stress–coping and behavioral choice models. Stress–coping models emphasize cognitive and behavioral coping responses that are available to individuals in the immediate high-risk situation for substance use.[46,47,53,54] For example, in Shiffman's research on smoking relapse,[46,47] the situational correlates of relapse and near relapse could be distinguished by whether or not former smokers reported having emitted either type of coping response. Although these findings suggest that the alternative responses that individuals emit in situations with substance cues influence their substance use outcomes, focusing on the immediate high-risk situation may neglect protective influences that operate over longer time periods. The treatment outcome findings discussed above point to the positive influence of more enduring components of individuals' life circumstances, and, to date, stress–coping accounts have not explicitly addressed the role of such influences.

The choice perspective, in contrast, is less concerned with individuals' responses in the immediate high-risk situation and focuses on the more molar aspects of individuals' ongoing life circumstances as they protect against or promote relapse. According to this view, the protective factors are seen as lying in the availability of alternative reinforcers to substance use that have minimal constraints on their access, and positive functioning during the posttreatment period is viewed as maintaining or increasing access to valued activities other than substance use. Although both the choice and stress–coping models share a general emphasis on the role of alternative behaviors in determining relapse and recovery, the choice perspective is less temporally constrained in its analysis of protective factors and thus is more easily integrated with the relevant treatment outcome findings.

Neither the dependence syndrome nor motivational models address this issue directly. Perhaps it could be inferred that low dependence protects against relapse, but without specification of the conditions that produce low dependence, this possibility is of little utility. With respect to motivational models, positive posttreatment functioning could be the result of fewer encounters with conditioned stimuli that activate the relevant motivational states; however, this possibility offers avoidance of the relevant cues as the only means of facilitating positive outcomes. Alternatively, positive functioning during the posttreatment period may somehow "block" the elicitation of the motivational states, even though the eliciting stimuli are encountered with the same frequency. Such a view, although conceptually coherent, still requires specification of the conditions that promote positive functioning.

Clinical Applications

Each of the four relapse models has generated applications aimed at characterizing the relapse process among clinical samples of substance abusers and/or developing relapse prevention strategies.

Dependence Syndrome Applications

Clinical research on the dependence syndrome has primarily addressed three issues:

1. Developing questionnaire measures of dependence[55–57];
2. Using dependence levels to differentiate substance abusers' responses to substance cues[21,22,58]; and
3. Using pretreatment dependence levels to predict treatment outcomes and to match clients in treatment to drinking goals of abstinence or moderation.[19,20,59]

The third line of research is most relevant to assessing the utility of the concept as a model of relapse.

Based on a review of alcohol studies that evaluated the relationship of alcohol dependence levels to treatment outcomes, Sobell and Sobell[13] concluded that the majority of supportive evidence derives from retrospective correlational analyses. More recent, prospective studies,[59,60] however, failed to find the predicted relationship between dependence and treatment outcomes and, as a result, Sobell and Sobell[13] concluded that "... the adoption of the obviously convenient ... severity of dependence tenet may have been premature" (p. 10). Instead, this work tentatively suggests that success with different drinking goals depends more on clients' beliefs about whether or not alcohol problems necessitate abstinence and, further, that allowing clients a choice of goals may facilitate positive outcomes, whether defined by abstinence or moderation drinking.[59,61,62] For example, Orford and Keddie[59] found that dependence levels did not affect clients' initial choice of moderation or abstinence goals or their drinking outcomes at 1-yr posttreatment. In contrast, positive treatment outcomes were facilitated when treatment orientation and initial goal assignment matched clients' beliefs about the nature of alcohol problems as either requiring abstinence or not.

Although these studies suggest that dependence levels do not provide a sound basis for treatment goal matching, other studies have found modest positive relationships between measures of dependence and treatment outcomes,[5,19] at least for male problem drinkers, with higher dependence being associated with higher relapse rates. This relationship is qualified, however, by other variables, including certain client characteristics and the circumstances that exist during the posttreatment interval. For example, Polich et al.[5] found complex interactions at 4 yr posttreatment between dependence levels, age, marital status, and clients' drinking status at an earlier follow-up point, and concluded that "both the environment and degree of dependence may affect the probability of relapse" (p. 176). In addition, the relationship of dependence levels to abstinence rates after treatment appears to vary with the length of follow-up. Studies that found higher dependence to be associated with higher relapse rates typically assessed outcomes during the first year after treatment,[19] whereas studies with follow-ups of 2 yr or more found that subjects who sustained long-term abstinence were characterized by relatively higher initial dependence.[5,63]

These findings tentatively suggest that higher dependence may make maintenance of abstinence more difficult during the early phase of the posttreatment interval, but that, in the absence of relapse-promoting environmental circumstances, higher dependence levels are not necessarily indicative of a poorer long-term prognosis. At a minimum, this pattern of results questions a simplistic application of the dependence syndrome to predict relapse after treatment that fails to consider the influence of client resources and characteristics of the posttreatment environment, as emphasized in other models of relapse. If the dependence syndrome model is to increase its utility in accounting for the relapse process, it must better specify how dependence levels moderate the demonstrated influence of other individual difference and environmental variables that are known to affect long-term drinking outcomes. Conceivably, pretreatment measures of dependence may best be viewed as an efficient means of summarizing subjects' history of drinking problems along a limited set of largely biological dimensions. Although higher dependence may indicate a general disposition to drink, the actions that constitute the disposition will only be manifested under certain conditions.[64] Discovery of those conditions remains a critical question in accounting for the relapse and recovery process, and, to date, the other three models of relapse have paid considerably more attention to delineating the relevant contextual variables.

Stress–Coping Applications

Clinical applications of this approach have focused on developing interventions aimed at relapse prevention (RP) after treatment.[27,28] A basic assumption of RP strategies is that clients will unavoidably encounter multiple substance cues and high-risk situations in their posttreatment environments. Therefore, RP strategies focus on training the skills necessary to deal effectively with the emotions, cognitions, and situations associated with past substance use and on minimizing the extent of substance use when it occurs. Central features of the approach are maintaining a nonjudgmental attitude when substance use occurs and viewing the episodes as important learning opportunities.

Marlatt's[28] RP program includes cognitive restructuring procedures designed to reduce the abstinence violation effect hypothesized to occur after initial substance use (*see* earlier section on Stress–Coping Models). In addition to these procedures aimed at limiting relapse severity, the program also includes elements of behavioral self-control treatments and related skills training treatments for addictive behaviors, such as self-monitoring of substance use urges and episodes of use, changing the topography of substance use behaviors to decrease use and intoxication levels, self-reinforcement of alternative responses to substance use, and role-playing substance refusal and adaptive coping responses. Although Marlatt's approach has exerted great influence on clinical approaches to relapse prevention during the past decade, its empirical support has not been consistent.[65–67] However, evaluation studies with negative findings often combined the RP program with other treatment components that were conceptually unrelated (e.g., more traditional interventions). Such combinations may have been confusing to clients or may have diluted the effects of the RP strategies, and comparisons of the effectiveness of RP alone in relation to other interventions are needed.[65]

Annis and colleagues[27,68] also have developed a RP program that emphasizes the role of efficacy expectations in preventing relapse in high-risk situations. Using Marlatt's[16] classification scheme of relapse determinants, Annis developed the Inventory of Drinking Situations (IDS), a self-report measure that assesses the extent to which alcohol use during the past year was associated with eight situational categories (e.g., social pressure to drink, unpleasant emotions). The IDS is then used to develop a hierarchy of risk situations for each client. Treatment involves progressive in vivo exposure to the situations, from low- to high-risk, a procedure designed to increase clients' self-efficacy expectations for avoiding substance use in the situations. Clients' coping skills in the high-risk situations also are assessed, for purposes of facilitating development of a wide array of adaptive responses. Although outcome evaluations of the approach currently are limited to those conducted by Annis and colleagues, the results obtained are encouraging and suggest that the IDS may provide an effective means for treatment matching. In a 6-mo follow-up study[68] that compared the effects of RP with more traditional counseling, clients who initially had differentiated IDS profiles, indicating variability in past drinking practices across situations, obtained better outcomes with the RP treatment than with the traditional treatment. For clients with generalized IDS profiles, no significant differences were found as a function of the type of treatment received.

In addition to the preliminary support obtained for specific RP programs, many of the cognitive–behavioral interventions included in the programs (e.g., social skills training, drink refusal training) have been favorably evaluated in general treatment outcome research.[69,70] Together, this work suggests that with further refinements in application, the relapse prevention approach holds much promise as a method of enhancing positive long-term outcomes.

Motivational–Conditioning Applications

If, as held by motivational–conditioning models, stimuli associated with past drug use or withdrawal function as conditioned stimuli for further substance use, then interventions aimed at extinguishing the conditioned responses may be beneficial. This approach has been widely used in treating anxiety and obsessive–compulsive disorders[71] and involves exposing clients to conditioned stimuli and preventing them from engaging in the problem behavior. As applied to substance disorders, clients are exposed to substance cues, such as the sight and smell of alcohol or drugs or the administration of an initial dose, and they are prevented or strongly discouraged from engaging in substance use. With repeated exposure that is followed by sustained abstinence, the eliciting properties of the stimuli should be extinguished, and clients should be better able to avoid substance use when the stimuli are encountered in their natural environments.

Cue exposure–response prevention treatments have been used with opiate addicts[72–74] with some success. However, including drug injections as part of the exposure component produced high rates of client attrition,[73] whereas use of a graduated hierarchy of drug-related stimuli, with optional self-injections, resulted in lower attrition rates.[72] The approach has been widely entertained as a viable treatment for alcohol problems, but research to date has not reported long-term follow-up data.[21,22] Until the effects of cue exposure–response prevention procedures on long-term outcomes are better evaluated, the utility of the approach must be considered undecided, especially as applied to alcohol abuse.

Behavioral Choice Applications

Clinical applications of the choice perspective are quite limited, perhaps because of the recency of the approach.[41,42] Nevertheless, a large experimental literature[41] that manipulated the constraints on access to alcohol and drugs and/or alternative reinforcers has supported the predicted effects on alcohol and drug self-administration, with substance use decreasing with increased constraints on substance access and increasing with increased constraints on alternative rewards. Importantly, a subset of these supportive experiments were conducted with human subjects with addictive disorders, including adult alcoholics,[75,76] drug abusers,[77] smokers,[78] and obese children.[79,80]

To our knowledge, the clinical implications of the choice perspective for relapse in the natural environment have only been directly investigated in our research on alcoholic relapse.[41,42,81] As mentioned earlier, one study of the first 6 mo after posttreatment[42] found that drinking episodes associated with events were more severe than those associated only with the immediate availability of alcohol; although guided by a different conceptual model, O'Connell and Martin[43] found a similar relationship regarding relapse severity in smokers. Also, in Vuchinich and Tucker's study,[42] events related to the life-health areas (e.g., family relationships, vocational functioning) that had been disrupted by subjects' past alcohol consumption were more likely to precipitate a relapse than those associated with events that had no prior contingent relationship with drinking problems. Both of these findings are consistent with this approach and suggest that pretreatment measures of the contingencies established between subjects' drinking and their access to rewards in important areas of functioning have value in predicting which posttreatment events are more likely to precipitate drinking in individual subjects. Although the implications for relapse prevention interventions have not yet been explored, this approach provides a means of identifying high-risk contexts prior to treatment initiation or termination for individual clients.

Another study[81] was aimed at characterizing the reinforcement value of alcohol relative to other activities during the pretreatment interval for use as a basis for predicting posttreatment relapse. Characterizing reinforcement value necessitates a measurement system that allows comparisons of individuals' behavioral allocation among qualitatively different activities that vary in the amount of resource (in terms of the response requirement, time, or money) required to gain access to each alternative. Since money is a basic and measurable human resource, it was used in this study to represent the relative reinforcement value of activities available to subjects during the pretreatment interval, including alcohol consumption. While hospitalized, alcoholics were interviewed about the amounts of income that they had allocated during the pretreatment year to different commodity classes (e.g., housing, food, entertainment), including alcohol consumption. The proportion of pretreatment monetary expenditure allocated to alcoholic beverages was positively related to drinking after treatment and was a better predictor of short-term outcomes than were measures of pretreatment drinking practices or demographic variables. If developed further, such an approach may provide a way to assess the severity of substance disorders that is independent of quantity–frequency measures of substance use, and may prove useful for treatment planning and treatment matching.

In addition to this preliminary work that supports analysis of the relapse process from the choice perspective, studies of the effectiveness of contingency management treatments also provide indirect support for the approach. A key component of contingency management is arranging differential consequences that discourage substance use and that reward alternative activities, which is consistent with the choice perspective. Contingency management has been found to be the treatment of choice for drug abuse[82] and is a central feature of the highly successful community reinforcement approach for treating alcoholics.[83]

Overall, this work supports the choice perspective as a conceptual framework for the relapse process and for impulsive behavior generally. Its several implications for the development of clinical assessment and intervention procedures appear to warrant further research attention.

Summary and Conclusions

Several conclusions emerge from this review. First, the dependence syndrome account of the relapse process is less comprehensive than the other three models. Although dependence may play a role in long-term substance use outcomes, its influence is probably more circumscribed than originally hypothesized. Moreover, the approach fails to address the known influence of environmental and other client resource variables on long-term treatment outcomes, an issue that is incorporated more easily into the other three approaches.

Second, of the remaining three models of relapse, all were found to address the three critical questions about the relapse process (*see* earlier in this chapter) and to provide a reasonable account of the observed relationship between posttreatment substance use and certain aspects of the surrounding environment. Important differences exist among the models, however, concerning the relevant properties of the environment, how they affect substance use, and the level of analysis of environment–relapse relationships. Until future research suggests otherwise, it probably is justified to view each of the three models as best addressing a subset of variables that influence the complex process of relapse and recovery after treatment. For example, stress–coping models offer a coherent framework for characterizing the interplay of relapse-risk and relapse-protective factors that are cast primarily in cognitive and affective terms and that operate in the immediate high-risk situation for substance use. Motivational–conditioning accounts, although also concerned with the immediate drug-taking environment, are better suited to conceptualizing how substance-related cues may exert an influcncc on individuals' current probability of drug use. Unlike the stress–coping and motivational approaches, the behavioral choice model adopts a more molar perspective on the temporal dynamics of the relapse process and emphasizes the contextual dependency of substance use in relation to changing constraints on other available activities. Because molecular and molar variables that operate over differing time frames probably combine to influence the probability of substance use at any point in time, both levels of analysis probably are important and likely have as yet unarticulated complementary relationships with one another.

Third, only two of the models, the stress–coping and choice accounts, directly address relapse-protective factors. Both emphasize the importance of alternative behaviors to substance use in relapse prevention, although the level of analysis is different. Stress–coping models focus on coping responses emitted in the immediate high-risk situation, and the choice model focuses on more enduring aspects of individuals' functioning in multiple life–health areas. Again, both types of alternatives probably are influential in promoting successful outcomes.

Fourth, with respect to the utility of the models in guiding clinical applications, except for research on the dependence syndrome, there has been insufficient work to warrant firm conclusions about the likely value of each of the other three models. Some support was found for key applications of all three models, and all yield promising implications for conceptualizing and intervening in the relapse process. However, none have been investigated thoroughly, especially those clinical applications derived from the motivational and choice perspectives. Relapse prevention programs of the stress–coping perspective have received more research attention, but it too is limited and, as noted earlier, may have been inadequate to evaluate the effectiveness of Marlatt's relapse prevention program apart from other treatment components.

Finally, even if well supported clinical assessment and/or intervention procedures are developed from any of the models of relapse, the difficult task of transferring this technology into widespread clinical use will remain. It has proven extremely difficult in the substance abuse field to influence clinical practice with data-based innovations. Despite several decades of research that fails to support disease-oriented models and treatments, this approach remains firmly entrenched in both the self-help and professional practice communities. Possible reasons for this situation have been widely discussed,[85–87] including the consistency of disease model approaches with the physician-dominated health-care delivery systems of which substance abuse treatment is now a part. Similarly, some have speculated that the rapid acceptance of the dependence syndrome model is due to its similarity to the disease model.[25,26] Based on the growing evidence questioning key assumptions of the model, including its application to relapse, we would agree with others[13,24,26] that continued emphasis cannot be justified scientifically.

In the short run, however, perhaps our goals for influencing clinical practice should be more modest. A major theme that has emerged from the literature on relapse and that seems to be gaining clinical acceptance is that some posttreatment substance use is common among treated clients and cannot be ignored in the treatment process. Traditional disease-oriented treatments do not directly address the relapse problem, but instead seek to promote continuous abstinence by offering substance abusers fellowship and support and an internally consistent framework for understanding their substance use as a disease beyond their control. This provides recovering addicts little guidance about how to minimize substance use episodes when they inevitably occur or a necessary understanding that a relapse episode need not result in a recovery failure.

Although we cannot cite supporting data, it is our impression that the value of relapse prevention is gaining a toehold within the clinical practice community. This is no small accomplishment given longstanding resistance to incorporating data-based treatments into clinical practice. Further acceptance of clinical applications derived from the relapse models will probably depend on their continued refinement, on demonstrations of their effectiveness, as well as on research aimed at facilitating effective technology transfer. Existing treatments may have yielded all that they can by way of reducing the relapse problem, and further improvements in long-term recovery rates are likely to come from a better understanding of the relapse and recovery process in the environments in which it occurs.

References

[1]J. Grabowski, M. L. Stitzer, and J. E. Henningfield (eds.) (1984) *Behavioral Intervention Techniques in Drug Abuse Treatment* (NIDA Research Monograph 46). US Government Printing Office, Washington, DC.

[2]W. R. Miller and R. K. Hester (1986) The effectiveness of alcoholism treatment, in *Treating Addictive Behaviors: Processes of Change*. W. R. Miller and R. K. Hester, eds. Plenum, New York, pp. 121–174.

[3]W. R. Miller and R. K. Hester (1986) Inpatient alcoholism treatment: Who benefits? *Am. Psychol.* **41,** 794–805.

[4]R. H. Moos, J. W. Finney, and R. C. Cronkite (1990) *Alcoholism Treatment: Context, Process, and Outcome*. Oxford University Press, New York.

[5]J. M. Polich, D. J. Armor, and H. B. Braiker (1981) *The Course of Alcoholism: Four Years After Treatment*. Wiley, New York.

[6]S. Shiffman (1992) Relapse process and relapse prevention in addictive behaviors. *Behav. Therapist* **15,** 9–11.

[7]J. A. Tucker (1992) Clinical research on addictive behaviors in the 1980's: Shifting focus from treatment outcome evaluations to studies of behavioral process. *Behav. Therapist* **15,** 4,5.

[8]K. D. Brownell, G. A. Marlatt, E. Lichtenstein, and G. T. Wilson (1986) Understanding and preventing relapse. *Am. Psychol.* **41,** 765–782.

[9]E. M. Pattison, M. B. Sobell, and L. C. Sobell (1977) *Emerging Concepts of Alcohol Dependence*. Springer, New York.

[10]N. K. Mello and J. H. Mendelson (1965) Operant analysis of drinking patterns of chronic alcoholics. *Nature* **206,** 43–46.

[11]G. A. Marlatt, B. Demming, and J. B. Reid (1973) Loss of control drinking in alcoholics: An experimental analogue. *J. Abnorm. Psychol.* **81,** 233–241.

[12]D. L. Davies (1962) Normal drinking in recovered alcohol addicts. *Q. J. Stud. Alcohol* **23,** 94–104.

[13]M. B. Sobell and L. C. Sobell (1987) Conceptual issues regarding goals in the treatment of alcohol problems. *Drugs Society* **1/2,** 1–37.

[14]J. R. Robertson, A. B. V. Bucknall, C. A. Skidmore, J. J. K. Roberts, and J. H. Smith (1989) Remission and relapse in heroin users and implications for management: Treatment control or risk reduction. *Int. J. Addict.* **24,** 229–246.

[15]S. Shiffman (1989) Tobacco "chippers": Individual differences in tobacco dependence. *Psychopharmacology* **91,** 539–547.

[16]G. A. Marlatt (1978) Craving for alcohol, loss of control, and relapse: A cognitive-behavioral analysis, in *Alcoholism: New Directions in Behavioral Research and Treatment* P. E. Nathan, G. A. Marlatt, and T. Loberg, eds. Plenum, New York, pp. 271–314.

[17]G. Edwards (1977) The alcohol dependence syndrome: Usefulness of an idea, in *Alcoholism: New Knowledge and New Responses.* G. Edwards and M. Grant, eds., University Park Press, London, pp. 136–156.

[18]G. Edwards, M. M. Gross, M. Keller, and J. Moser (eds.) (1976) Alcohol-related problems in the disability perspective. A summary of the consensus of the WHO group of investigators on criteria for identifying and classifying disabilities related to alcohol consumption. *Q. J. Stud. Alcohol* **9,** 1360–1382.

[19]T. F. Babor, N. L. Cooney, and R. J. Lauerman (1987) The dependence syndrome concept as a psychological theory of relapse behaviour: An empirical evaluation of alcoholic and opiate addicts. *Br. J. Addict.* **82,** 393–405.

[20]N. Heather, S. Rollnick, and M. Winton (1983) A comparison of objective and subjective measures of alcohol dependence as predictors of relapse following treatment. *Br. J. Clin. Psychol.* **22,** 11–17.

[21]H. Rankin, R. Hodgson, and T. Stockwell (1980) The behavioural measurement of dependence. *Br. J. Addict.* **75,** 43–47.

[22]H. Rankin, R. Hodgson, and T. Stockwell (1983) Cue exposure and response prevention with alcoholics: A controlled trial. *Behav. Res. Ther.* **21,** 435–446.

[23]T. F. Babor (1986) Comments on Griffith Edwards' 'The alcohol dependence syndrome: Concept as a stimulus to enquiry'—1. Philosophical and scientific issues. *Br. J. Addict.* **81,** 185–187.

[24]I. Robertson (1986) Comments on Griffith Edwards' 'The alcohol dependence syndrome: Concept as a stimlus to enquiry'—3. A modest statistical phenomenon of little theoretical coherence. *Br. J. Addict.* **81,** 190–193.

[25]S. Shaw (1980) A critique of the concept of the alcohol dependence syndrome. *Br. J. Addict.* **74,** 339–348.

[26]S. Shaw (1985) The disease concept of dependence, in *The Misuse of Alcohol; Crucial Issues in Dependence, Treatment, and Prevention.* N. Heather, I. Robertson, P. Davies, eds. Croom Helm, London, pp. 35–44.

[27]H. M. Annis and C. S. Davis (1989) Relapse prevention, in *Handbook of Alcoholism Treatment: Effective Alternatives.* R. K. Hester and W. R. Miller, eds. Pergamon, New York, pp. 170–182.

[28]G. A. Marlatt and J. R. Gordon (eds.) (1985) *Relapse Prevention.* Guilford, New York.

[29]S. Shiffman (1989) Conceptual issues in the study of relapse, in *Relapse and Addictive Behaviour*. M. Gossop, ed. Croom Helm, Kent, England, pp. 149–179.

[30]R. S. Lazarus (1966) *Psychological Stress and the Coping Process.* Appleton-Century-Crofts, New York.

[31]M. M. Condiotte and E. Lichtenstein (1981) Self-efficacy and relapse in smoking cessation programs. *J. Consult. Clin. Psychol.* **49,** 648–658.

[32]C. C. DiClemente (1981) Self-efficacy and smoking cessation maintenance: A preliminary report. *Cognitive Ther. Res.* **5,** 175–187.

[33]J. A. Tucker, R. E. Vuchinich, and C. V. Harris (1985) Determinants of substance abuse relapse, in *Determinants of Substance Abuse: Biological, Psychological, and Environmental Factors.* M. Galizio and S. A. Maisto, eds. Plenum, New York, pp. 383–421.

[34]J. A. Tucker, R. E. Vuchinich, and A. J. Gladsjo (1990/91) Environmental influences on relapse in substance use disorders. *Int. J. Addict.* **25,** 1017–1050.

[35]T. B. Baker, E. Morse, and J. E. Sherman (1987) The motivation to use drugs: A psychobiological analysis of urges, in *Nebraska Symposium on Motivation: Alcohol and Addictive Behavior.* P. C. Rivers, ed. University of Nebraska Press, Lincoln, NE, pp. 257–323.

[36]A. M. Ludwig and A. Wikler (1974) "Craving" and relapse to drink. *Q. J. Stud. Alcohol* **35,** 108–130.

[37]R. S. Niaura, D. J. Rohsenow, J. A. Binkoff, P. M. Monti, M. Pedraza, and D. B. Abrams (1988) Relevance of cue reactivity to understanding alcohol and smoking relapse. *J. Abnorm. Psychol.* **97,** 133–152.

[38]J. Stewart, H. de Wit, and R. Eikelboom (1984) Role of conditioned and unconditioned drug effects in the self-administration of opiates and stimulants. *Psychol. Rev.* **91,** 251-268.

[39]H. Rachlin, R. Battalio, J. Kagel, and L. Green (1981) Maximization theory in behavioral psychology. *Behav. Brain Sci.* **4,** 371–417.

[40]R. J. Herrnstein (1971) On the law of effect. *J. Exp. Analysis Behav.* **13,** 243–266.

[41]R. E. Vuchinich and J. A. Tucker (1988) Contributions from behavioral theories of choice to an analysis of alcohol abuse. *J. Abnorm. Psychol.* **97,** 181–195.

[42]R. E. Vuchinich and J. A. Tucker (1991) Relapse in alcoholics as choice behavior. Unpublished manuscript, Auburn University.

[43]K. A. O'Connell and E. J. Martin (1987) Highly tempting situations associated with abstinence, temporary lapse, and relapse among participants in smoking cessation programs. *J. Consult. Clin. Psychol.* **55,** 367–371.

[44]H. Skinner (1986) Comments on Griffith Edwards' 'The alcohol dependence syndrome: Concept as a stimulus to enquiry'—4. Alcohol dependence: How does it come about? *Br. J. Addict.* **81,** 193–196.

[45]B. D. Hore (1971) Life events and alcoholic relapse. *Br. J. Addict.* **6,** 25–37.

[46]S. Shiffman (1982) Relapse following smoking cessation: A situational analysis. *J. Consult. Clin. Psychol.* **50,** 71–86.

[47]S. Shiffman (1984) Coping with temptations to smoke. *J. Consult. Clin. Psychol.* **52,** 261–267.

[48]H. Lei and H. A. Skinner (1980) A psychometric study of life events and social readjustment. *J. Psychosom. Res.* **24,** 57–65.

[49]J. D. Hawkins and M. W. Frazer (1987) The social networks of drug abusers before and after treatment. *Int. J. Addict.* **22,** 343–355.

[50]R. Mermelstein, S. Cohen, E. Lichtenstein, J. S. Baer, and T. Kamarck (1986) Social support and smoking cessation and maintenance. *J. Consult. Clin. Psychol.* **554,** 447–453.

[51]S. A. Maisto and J. B. McCollam (1980) The use of multiple measures of life health to assess alcohol treatment outcome: A review and critique, in *Evaluating Alcohol and Drug Abuse Treatment Effectiveness.* L. C. Sobell, M. B. Sobell, and E. Ward, eds. Pergamon, New York, pp. 15–76.

[52]W. R. Miller, K. E. Hedrick, and C. A. Taylor (1983) Addictive behaviors and life problems before and after behavioral treatment of problem drinkers. *Addict. Behav.* **8,** 403–412.

[53]A. G. Billings and R. H. Moos (1983) Psychosocial processes of recovery among alcoholics and their families: Implications for clinicians and program evaluators. *Addict. Behav.* **8,** 205–218.

[54]M. E. Wewers (1988) The role of postcessation events in tobacco abstinence, stressful events and coping responses. *Addict. Behav.* **13,** 297–302.

[55]R. Davidson (1987) Assessment of the alcohol dependence syndrome: A review of self-report screening questionnaires. *Br. J. Clin. Psychol.* **26,** 243–255.

[56]H. A. Skinner and B. A. Allen (1982) Alcohol dependence syndrome: Measurement and validation. *J. Abnorm. Psychol.* **91,** 199–209.

[57]T. Stockwell, D. Murphy, and R. Hodgson (1983) The severity of alcohol dependence questionnaire: Its use, reliability and validity. *Br. J. Addict.* **78,** 145–155.

[58]H. Rankin, T. Stockwell, and R. Hodgson (1982) Cues for drinking and degrees of alcohol dependence. *Br. J. Addict.* **77,** 287–296.

[59]J. Orford and A. Keddie (1986) Abstinence or controlled drinking in clinical practice: A test of the dependence and persuasion hypotheses. *Br. J. Addict.* **81,** 495–504.

[60]G. Elal-lawrence, P. D. Slade, and M. E. Dewey (1986) Predictors of outcome type in treated problem drinkers. *J. Stud. Alcohol* **47,** 41–47.

[61]W. R. Miller and R. K. Hester (1986) Matching problem drinkers with optimal treatments, in *Treating Addictive Behaviors: Processes of Change.* W. R. Miller and R. K. Hester, eds. Plenum, New York, pp. 175–203.

[62]M. Sanchez-Craig and D. A. Wilkinson (1987) Treating problem drinkers who are not severely dependent on alcohol. *Drugs Society* **1/2,** 39–67.

[63]J. Orford, E. Oppenheimer, and G. Edwards (1976) Abstinence or control: The outcome for excessive drinkers two years after consultation. *Behav. Res. Ther.* **14,** 409–418.

[64]R. E. Vuchinich (1991) The context dependence of alcoholic relapse. Paper

presented at the meeting of the Research Society on Alcoholism, Marco Island, FL, June.

[65]S. J. Curry, G. A. Marlatt, J. Gordon, and J. S. Baer (1988) A comparison of alternative theoretical approaches to smoking cessation and relapse. *Health Psychol.* **7,** 545–556.

[66]S. M. Hall, D. Rugg, C. Tunstall, and R. T. Jones (1984) Preventing relapse to cigarette smoking by behavioral skill training. *J. Consult. Clin. Psychol.* **52,** 372–382.

[67]J. R. Ito, D. M. Donovan, and J. J. Hall (1988) Relapse prevention in alcohol aftercare: Effects on drinking outcome, change process, and aftercare compliance in alcoholic veterans. *Br. J. Addict.* **83,** 171–181.

[68]H. M. Annis, C. S. Davis, M. Graham, and T. A. Levinson. A controlled trial of relapse prevention procedures based on self-efficacy theory. Unpublished manuscript, Addiction Research Foundation, Toronto.

[69]E. F. Chaney, M. R. O'Leary, and G. A. Marlatt (1978) Skill training with alcoholics. *J. Consult. Clin. Psychol.* **46,** 1092–1104.

[70]P. M. Monti, D. B. Abrams, R. M. Kadden, and N. L. Cooney (1989) *Treating Alcohol Dependence*. Guilford, New York.

[71]E. B. Foa and M. J. Kozak (1986) Emotional processing of fear: Exposure to corrective information. *Psychol. Bull.* **99,** 20–35.

[72]A. R. Childress, A. T. McClellan, and C. P. O'Brien (1985) Assessment and extinction of conditioned wihtdrawal-like responses in an integrated treatment for opiate dependence, in *Problems of Drug Dependence, 1984* (NIDA Research Monograph 55). L. S. Harris, ed., US Government Printing Office, Washington, DC, pp. 202–210.

[73]C. P. O'Brien, R. Ehrman, and J. Ternes (1986) Classical conditioning in human opioid dependence, in *Behavioral Analysis of Drug Dependence*. S. R. Goldberg and I. P. Stolerman, eds. Academic, Orlando, FL, pp. 329–356.

[74]C. P. O'Brien, R. Greenstein, J. Ternes, T. McLellan, and J. Grabowski (1979) Unreinforced self-injections: Effects of rituals and outcome in heroin addicts, in *Problems of Drug Dependence, 1979* (NIDA Research Monograph 27). L. S. Harris, ed. U.S. Government Printing Office, Washington, DC, pp. 275–281.

[75]M. Cohen, I. A. Liebson, and L. A. Faillance (1971) The modification of drinking of chronic alcoholics, in *Recent Advances in Studies of Alcoholism*. N. K. Mello and J. H. Mendelson, eds. US Government Printing Office, Washington, DC, pp. 745–766.

[76]R. R. Griffiths, G. E. Bigelow, and I. Liebson (1978) Relationship of social factors to ethanol: Self-administration in alcoholics, in *Alcoholism: New Directions in Behavioral Research and Treatment*. P. E. Nathan, G. A. Marlatt, and T. Loberg, eds. Plenum, New York, pp. 351–380.

[77]M. L. Stitzer, G. E. Bigelow, and I. Liebson (1979) Reinforcement of drug

abstinence: A behavioral approach to drug abuse treatment, in *Behavioral Analysis and Treatment of Substance Abuse* (NIDA Research Monograph 25). N. Krasner, ed. US Government Printing Office, Washington, DC, pp. 65–90.

[78]L. H. Epstein, C. M. Bulik, K. A. Perkins, A. R. Caggiula, and J. Rodefer (1991) Behavioral economic analysis of smoking: Money and food as alternatives. *Pharmacol. Biochem. Behav.* **38,** 1–7.

[79]L. H. Epstein, J. A. Smith, L. S. Vara, and J. S. Rodefer (1991) Behavioral economic analysis of activity choice in obese children. *Health Psychol.* **10,** 311–316.

[80]J. A. Smith and L. H. Epstein (in press) Behavioral economic analysis of food choice in obese children. *Appetite.*

[81]R. E. Vuchinich and J. A. Tucker (1987) Predicting alcoholic relapse with pretreatment measures of drinking behavior and money spent on drinking. Paper presented at the Conference on Experimental and Behavioral Approaches to Alcoholism, Bergin, Norway, August.

[82]G. E. Bigelow, M. L. Stitzer, and I. Liebson (1984) The role of behavioral contingency management in drug abuse, in *Behavioral Intervention Techniques in Drug Abuse Treatment.* (NIDA Research Monograph 46). J. Grabowski, M. L. Stitzer, and J. E. Henningfield, eds. U.S. Government Printing Office Washington, DC, pp. 36–52.

[83]R. W. Sisson and N. H. Azrin (1989) The community reinforcement approach, in R. K. Hester, W. R. Miller, eds. *Handbook of Alcoholism Treatment Approaches: Effective Alternatives.* Pergamon, New York, pp. 242–258.

[84]G. A. Marlatt (1987) Research and political realities: What the next twenty years hold for behaviorists in the alcohol field. *Adv. Behav. Res. Ther.* **9,** 165–171.

[85]W. R. Miller (1987) Behavioral alcohol treatment advances: Barriers to utilization. *Adv. Behav. Res. Ther.* **9,** 145–164.

[86]M. B. Sobell and L. C. Sobell (1984) The aftermath of heresay: A response to Pendery et al.'s critique of "Individualized Behavior for Alcoholics." *Behav. Res. Ther.* **22,** 412–440.

[87]J. A. Tucker, R. E. Vuchinich, and K. K. Downey (1992) Substance abuse, in *Handbook of Clinical Behavior Therapy,* (2nd ed.). S. M. Turner, K. S. Calhoun, and H. E. Adams, eds. Wiley, New York, pp. 203–223.

Charting the Psychological Correlates of Drug Abuse

Lorand B. Szalay, Shelley K. Vilov, and Jean B. Strohl

Introduction

Limited Success in Relating Drug Use and Personality

For decades, researchers interested in the psychological dimensions of drug use have focused primarily on personality traits. They assumed that psychological effects of habitual drug use may be best identified by measuring changes in relevant personality traits. Since this approach followed, rather naturally, from the high status of personality constructs in psychology, the inconclusive findings of the research came as a surprise.

Consider, for example, one of the most researched personality traits: external vs internal locus of control. This was found to correlate significantly with substance abuse in some studies,[1–6] but not in others.[7–14] McBride suggested that such different results may be owing to test settings that elevate social desirability and thereby inflate internality scores.[14] Des Jarlais found that treatment represented a reassertion of lost control for heroin addicts, suggesting that locus of control is situationally influenced.[9] Right or wrong, the fact remains that studies on this trait do not consistently support broader generalizations.

From: *Drug and Alcohol Abuse Reviews, Vol. 4: Drug Abuse Treatment*
Ed: R. R. Watson ©1992 The Humana Press Inc.

In a recent review of personality concepts and their relationship to addiction, Sutker and Allian concluded that the etiology, expression, and consequences of substance abuse require broader conceptualizations that encompass biological and sociocultural dimensions in addition to personological dimensions.[15] Although researchers vary in their conclusions, they show a similar trend in shifting their focus of attention away from personality constructs.

Another line of research has followed background variables and social attitudes such as alienation. Again, results are mixed. Alienation was found to be associated with substance abuse in some populations[16–20] but not in others.[21,22] Furthermore, alienation has been significantly correlated with the use of some drugs, but this correlation has been weak and of no explanatory value with regard to the use of other drugs.[23,24] Concomitant variables may contribute to the weak association between alienation and substance abuse. For example, both drug use and alienation have been predicted by extroversion, fluid intelligence, lack of acculturation, and independence.[25] The inconsistency in the relationship of alienation and substance abuse may also be owing in part to varied conceptions of alienation, such as powerlessness, social isolation, and normative ambiguity.

Social alienation, similar to most personality constructs, is a complex variable approached through a variety of concepts and measures. These differences in the general concept of alienation account for much of the apparently contradictory findings and limit the use of these constructs to produce generalizable results on the psychological aspects of drug use.

Rather than using high level constructs of questionable applicability, the approach used in this research relies on the identification of perceptions and evaluations that differentiate drug users and nonusers. It maps trends in the organization of mental representations along dimensions related to drug use such as self image, social relations, and subjective views of harmful substances.

Approach: Focus on Perceptions and Mental Representations

The approach relies on an analytic assessment that works by reconstructing perceptions and evaluations as mosaic pieces of subjective images and meanings. These are obtained empirically from the distribution of thousands of spontaneous free associations. Although an approach based on free associations and designed to map subjective images and meanings could create the impression of being divorced from behavior, the results reported here show that it is possible to differentiate users and nonusers with a high degree of accuracy by charting systems of mental representations. Cognitive theorists have long assumed an intimate relationship between mental representations and behavior, but an empirical demonstration of this relationship was hampered by the limitations of the more direct and structured methods of assessment.

Students of human behavior working along theories of cognitive representation assume that much of goal-oriented human behavior is guided by cognitive maps of systems of mental representation. Triandis spoke of a system of cognitions that constitutes a map of the ways people conceive their environment.[26] Tolman described the maps as guidance or control systems that exert continuous influences on choices and behavior.[27] Models of mental representations include such diverse notions as cognitive map,[27] cognitive representation,[28] internal representation,[29,30] subjective lexicon,[31] meaningful system,[32] and thought world.[33] These converge in their fundamental assumptions that people's behavior is organized and guided by their subjective meanings, by the system of subjective views they develop in the representation of their subjective world.

We speak here purposefully of subjective representations rather than of beliefs and opinions. This is to underscore that opinions and beliefs are, for the most part, conscious positions assumed by people who are mostly aware of their subjective choices. As our in-depth studies of various cultures have shown, however, subjective images and meanings are experienced and held by people as the simple, unadulterated representation of reality. This sensation that they represent plain and simple reality explains why they are so resistant to change and why they constitute such persistent barriers to human understanding. Also, this sensation of representing plain realities is probably the key to the close control they exert on behavior.

Such considerations may also explain why, following the psychological tradition, the main thrust of empirical research designed to reconstruct systems of subjective representations is centered on the assessment of subjective images and meanings. Compared to lexical meanings based on linguistic use or convention, psychological meanings are subjective reactions[32] that frequently encompass affects, personal experiences, and perspectives. They constitute elementary units or mosaic pieces of the global system of mental representation or world view. The system of subjective representation is not merely an aggregate of subjective images and meanings but a highly organized, coherent system. These representational units are highly interdependent; each unit has to fit and be adapted by the system. The Associative Group Analysis method was used to assess subjective images and meanings as representational units and to reconstruct the main parameters of systems of mental representation.

Hypotheses

The research tested three main assumptions based on a representational model of behavioral organization.

1. Drug users and nonusers differ in their perceptions and evaluations that are identifiable and correlate significantly with drug use.
2. The perceptual and evaluative differences identified between users and nonusers reflect broad and consistent trends that reflect differences between two systems of subjective representations.
3. User and nonuser type perceptual and evaluative dispositions measured along various dimensions of subjective representations show positive correlations with actual drug use.

Method

Subjects

Over 2500 students were tested from eight colleges participating in a pilot study of prevention programs sponsored by the US Department of Education. The colleges participating in the research were chosen from a large pool of 200 colleges that received federal grant support for developing and implementing proactive drug prevention programs in the field of postsecondary education. Those included in the research represent a broad geographic distribution, both 2- and 4-year colleges, as well as private and state colleges. The analysis reported in this chapter is based on two samples of drug users and nonusers of comparable age, sex, and other sociodemographic characteristics.

1. Nonusers (n = 200): students who reported under conditions of strict anonymity that they have never used illicit drugs.
2. Frequent users (n = 200) students who reported that they used marijuana and/or other illicit drugs more frequently than once a month.

The AGA method was administered to the subjects using stimulus themes covering several domains: self concept, drug use, interpersonal and social relations, work, and future. The standard AGA data collection procedures were used to elicit multiple response, free associations to the selected themes.

Procedure

The Associative Group Analysis Method

The theoretical rationale of using word associations in the empirical study of meanings has its roots in the work of Noble[34] and Deese.[35] As described in the monograph *Subjective Meaning and Culture*,[36] the Associative Group Analysis (AGA) Method relies on continued free associations to reconstruct the subjective images and meanings of selected samples of respondents. AGA is a highly unstructured and open-ended analytical method. It offers access to behavioral dispositions beyond the reach of more direct and more structured methods of assessment. It does not call for an overt expression of personal position or opinions as no specific questions are asked. The respondents perceive association as a language task rather than an attempt to probe their personal beliefs or attitudes.

Data Collection, Test Administration

In its most common form, AGA uses association tasks administered in written form to selected samples in group sessions. They receive the word themes (e.g., ME) printed several times on slips of paper. They are asked to write as many ideas related to each theme presented as they can think of in 1 minute. On the average the participants give six to eight different associations to each word presented. As experiments have shown, the first responses are slightly more informative on the subjective meaning than the ones that follow. These differences have been measured experimentally by retesting the stability of responses at various rank places, and used to assign weight to the responses. The weights obtained are as follows: 6,5,4,3,3,3,3,2,2,1,1,1. The weighted responses produced by the members of a particular group (e.g., frequent drug users) are tallied into response distributions as shown in Table 1.

Mosaic Pieces of Perceptions and Evaluations

Table 1 presents some of the most frequent responses elicited by the stimulus theme marijuana by drug users and nonusers. Based on the distributions of hundreds of spontaneous responses, such response lists offer the main mosaic pieces of the respondents' subjective perceptions and

Table 1
Top-Ranking Responses to Marijuana by Frequent Users and Nonusers

Frequent users		Nonusers	
Response	Score	Response	Score
high	320	drug(s)	532
pot	311	smoke(ing)	281
smoke(ing)	291	bad	275
drug(s)	211	pot	256
joint(s)	183	illegal	232
fun	142	high	195
bong(s)	120	addiction	119
addiction	112	plant(s)	107
goodness	96	stupid(ity)	101
stone(d)	95	weed(s)	99
dope	86	joint(s)	73
bad	83	grass	70
weed(s)	78	cigaret(s)	64
green	70	danger(ous)	53
grass	69	dope	52
pipe(s)	67	harm(ful)	52
illegal	61	kill(ing)	49
money	58	money	49
relax(ation)	58	stone(d)	42
expensive	50	smell(ing)	41
Mary Jane	47	stink(ing)	38
reefer	47	death	38
party(s)	46	dumb	34
friend(s)	38	Mary Jane	32

evaluations. Each response has a score value. These values reveal how salient a particular idea or attribute is (fun, illegal) as a mosaic of the group's image of marijuana. A quick, perfunctory comparison of the responses suggests some characteristic differences in the way drug users and nonusers view marijuana. For instance, the drug users focus on the experience of getting high whereas the nonusers view marijuana as bad and illegal.

Because the mosaic pieces revealed by the response distributions are many and frequently related in natural clusters, several analytic procedures have been developed to arrive at more global and systematic

Table 2
Main Components of Perceptions and Evaluations of Marijuana
by Frequent Users and Nonusers

Main components	Percentage of total score	
	Users	Nonusers
Pot, grass, weed	20	17
Smoking, joint, smell	21	14
Effects: high, stoned	17	8
Fun, parties, good	11	2
Addiction, harmful, death	6	12
Bad,stupid	4	16
Illegal, police	4	9
Drugs, alcohol	8	15
Money, selling	4	3
Friends, school	2	4
Miscellaneous	2	1
Total scores	4284	4222

conclusions. A simple method involves content analysis. Analysts with backgrounds comparable to the respondents', trained in this process, group the responses into relevant clusters or categories. For instance, responses conveying negative affects are placed in one cluster labeled by the most salient reactions: bad, harmful. References to positive affects are placed in another cluster, labeled again by the highest scoring reactions: fun, good.

As past studies have shown, such categorizations or content analysis can be performed with a reasonable degree of reliability. The mean correlation between analysts working independently was .7. An application of this procedure to the responses of the drug users and nonusers to marijuana resulted in the main response clusters shown in Table 2. The drug users reveal their familiarity with the nature and use of marijuana: high, stoned, smoke, joint, bong. The users show predominantly positive attitudes, viewing marijuana as fun, good, relaxing. They pay less attention to negative evaluations and harmful consequences yet their responses do convey some ambivalence. The nonusers think of marijuana in more general terms, identifying it emphatically as a drug and rejecting it as bad, stupid, harmful, and dangerous. They show more concern with the legal consequences associated with its use. Although not apparent in Table 1, in the overall analysis nonusers think more of the role of dealers and pushers in promoting the use of marijuana.

To convey the summarized results in a simple visual form, we use "semantographs" (Fig. 1). The semantograph is a graphical presentation showing the differential salience of the main perceptual and evaluative components of each group's subjective image. The bars of the graph represent the main components of the group's image. On this graph the outlined bars show the relative salience of perceptions and attitudes of the frequent user group; the shaded bars show the salience of these same perceptual and attitudinal components for the nonuser group. This technique of visual presentation is used to offer a quick comparison useful in the identification of main similarities and differences. On a few select clusters where the differences appear sizable, the actual reactions of the groups are listed in detail.

Several analytic measures have been applied to gage the organization of the system along such main dimensions as priorities, perceptions, and evaluations.

Subjective Priorities, Importance

The importance of a particular stimulus theme to a particular person or group is inferred from the number of responses offered in the association task. The "dominance" scores calculated both on an individual and group basis are analogous to Noble's widely tested measure of "meaningfulness."[34] They have been used to measure differences between culture groups in their subjective priorities, as well as to trace changes in priorities over time. The reliability of the group dominance score ($r = .93$) was tested by test–retest comparison.[37] The individual dominance similarity scores used in this research show the dominance scores of each user and nonuser on each theme compared with dominance scores obtained from users and nonusers on a group basis.

Subjective Perceptions, Representations

The similarity of subjective views and perceptions of a particular theme for different groups can be measured by comparing the distributions of their free associations, using Pearson's measure of product–moment correlation. The test–retest reliability of this measure was around .9 in several investigations.[38] The individual perceptual similarity scores were

EFFECTS: HIGH, STONED	USR 744	NON 330
high, getting high	333	195
stone(d)	95	42
fly(ing)	11	—
escaping, release, relief	35	8
relax(ation)	58	9
out of control	—	9
wasted	—	7
buzz(ed)	11	—
paranoid, confused, dizzy	41	6
trip, hallucinate	14	—
hungry, munchies, food	50	9
sleep(ing), tired(ness)	24	—
brain(s)	—	31
alter(ing)	—	8
mood(-swing)	10	—
feel(ing)	9	—
comfort(ing)	5	—
peaceful, mellow, euphoria	30	—
carefree, free(dom)	18	6

FUN, PARTIES, GOOD	USR 475	NON 76
fun	142	12
laugh(ter)	24	8
party(s)	46	21
enjoy(ment)	21	—
good(ness), great(ness)	102	18
like, love, yes, ok	40	—
cool	25	—
sex(ual)	10	—
music, concerts	11	6
happy(ness)	9	7
drink(ing), drunk	3	4
want	6	—
entertain(ment)	8	—
excite(ment)	4	—
social(able)	7	—
quality(s)	8	—
intense(ity)	9	—

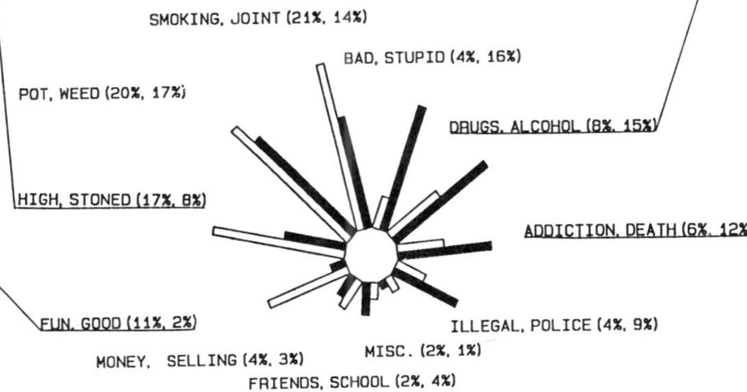

DRUGS, ALCOHOL	USR 326	NON 617
drug(s)	211	532
dope	86	52
beer	8	—
cocaine	21	7
alcohol	—	9
depressant(s)	—	9
stimulant	—	8

ADDICTION, HARMFUL, DEATH	USR 272	NON 523
addiction	112	119
addict(s)	6	19
habit(forming)	10	5
daily	9	—
harm,hurt,damage,destroy	33	109
danger(ous)	—	53
unhealthy	—	26
death, deadly	7	45
kill(ing)	9	49
sick(ness)	—	16
cough(ing)	6	8
lung(s)	13	—
accident	—	6
depression	9	—
downer(s)	12	—
fight(ing)	—	8
problem(s)	28	29
brain cells, brain-dead	8	18
burn out	10	—
abuse	—	13

Fig. 1. Perceptions and evaluations of marijuana by college drug users (▭, total score: 4284) and nonusers (▬, total score: 4222).

calculated by developing lists of responses that differentiate users and nonusers and using these lists to score individual respondents on whether their responses were more like the user group or the nonuser group.

Subjective Affects, Evaluations

As extensive attitude research has demonstrated, affects, positive vs negative evaluations, are important psychological variables. One of the ways to reconstruct how a person or group evaluates a particular stimulus theme is to calculate the predominance of positive vs negative responses to particular stimulus themes. The Evaluative Dominance Indices, calculated on the basis of positive vs negative reactions, produced very high positive correlations of .86–.90 with independent attitude measures (e.g., semantic differential evaluation factor scales).[39] In this study the attitudinal measure is calculated on an individual basis and used to isolate differences between users and nonusers.

Results

Drug users and nonusers were compared at three different levels: (1) specific views and attitudes differentiating users and nonusers on select variables like drugs and self-image; (2) perceptual and motivational dispositions observed across several themes for each group; (3) differences in the groups' systems of mental representation. We also wanted to test the utility of these perceptual and attitudinal results to identify user vs nonuser type dispositions that differentiate between people with different behavior.

Differences in the Subjective Images Characteristic of Drug Users and Nonusers

As units of mental representation, the subjective images of user and nonuser groups are compared to identify differences in their perceptions and attitudes. This process was illustrated with the example of marijuana and is further shown here in regard to two other drug-related themes.

The Image of Drugs

Although users think more about specific illicit drugs, they show relatively few negative evaluations compared to the nonusers. They relate drugs more to fun, party, and sex. Parallel to positive experiences and evaluations, users do show a concern with addiction and such negative consequences as death. Such ambivalence reveals a great deal of internal contradiction. Although this group thinks less about harmful consequences and illegality, the users' characterization of drugs as bad does reflect some strong negative feelings as well. Their meaning of drugs also includes the mind-altering effects of drug experiences like high, hallucination, and escape, which are not part of the nonuser's perception.

Nonusers pay more attention to the medical applications of drugs referring to doctors, prescriptions, and substances with medicinal effects. The more narrow meaning of drugs as illicit substances provokes more uniformly negative evaluations. Nonusers characterize drugs as bad, stupid, scary, and awful. They show intense concern with the harmful and dangerous effects of drugs such as addiction, death, and killing. They also show more concern with illegality and the legal consequences of using illicit drugs (*see* Fig. 2).

The Image of Alcohol

Users think more of specific types and brands of hard liquor and beer. Both the users and nonusers show similar concern with addiction and abuse, but the users place less emphasis on alcoholism, dependency, and addicts. On the other hand, they show more recognition of Alcoholics Anonymous. Users show more awareness of certain negative hangover effects such as throwing up and vomiting, indicating more direct personal experiences. They identify alcohol more with fun, happiness, and excitement, and associate it more with sex.

Nonusers are more negative, characterizing alcohol as bad and stupid. They think more about the habit-forming effects of alcohol use. Nonusers are much more concerned about the problem of drunk driving, emphasizing accidents, death, killing, and dangerous. They also identify health problems associated with alcohol use. The nonusers associate alcohol more with drugs (*see* Fig. 3).

Trends of Perceptions and Evaluations by Users and Nonusers Across Domains

"Drugs, Addiction" Domain

It is apparent from the findings obtained on marijuana, drugs, and alcohol that the users differ from nonusers along trends of perceptions and evaluations that emerge with considerable consistency. Across the themes used in the representation of the "Drug, Addiction" domain (marijuana, drugs, alcohol, and addiction), nonusers are very concerned about

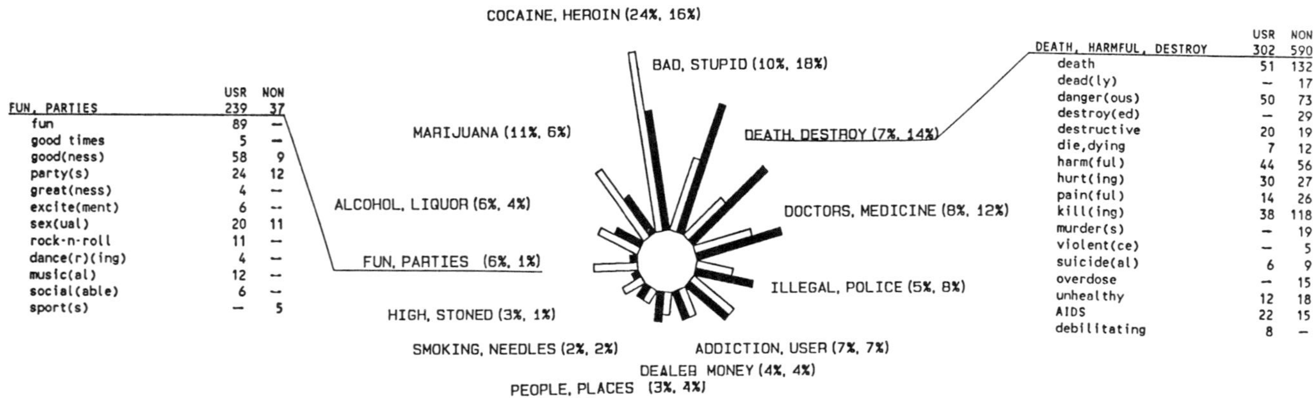

Fig. 2. Perceptions and evaluations of drugs by college drug users (▭, total score: 4148) and nonusers (■, total score: 4269).

FUN, GOOD, RELAXATION	USR 317	NON 192
fun	179	92
good times	17	8
good(ness)	33	45
like	—	5
relax(ation)	35	27
relief, release	4	15
enjoy(ment), pleasure	15	—
happy(ness)	15	—
excite(ment)	10	—
free(dom)	9	—

HANGOVER, SICK	USR 148	NON 100
hangover	42	42
sick(ness)	50	39
throwing up, vomiting	41	13
headache	9	6
stomach	6	—

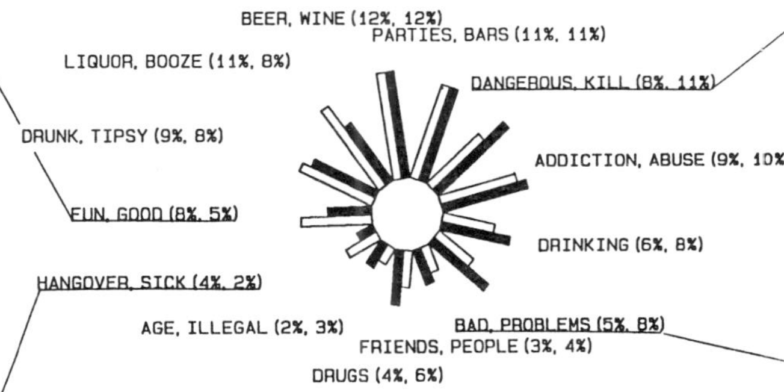

DANGEROUS, KILL, ACCIDENT	USR 347	NON 438
danger, ous	42	47
kill(ing)	32	47
death, deadly	52	66
drunk driving	8	22
drive(ing), cars	55	84
DWI, DUI	47	25
don't drive	11	11
accident, crash	23	38
destroy(ed)	—	8
hurting, harmful, pain	28	30
liver	15	20
poison(ing)	9	12
brain cells	—	6
violence, aggression, fight	25	22

BAD, PROBLEMS	USR 190	NON 345
bad	76	113
stupid, dumb, idiotic, foolish	8	43
problem(s)	41	35
depressant(s)	15	43
nasty, evil	—	24
unnecessary, not needed	—	18
hate(ful)	7	—
trouble, mess	14	19
helpless(ness)	4	—
unhealthy	—	22
sting(s)	4	—
sad, lonely, scared	21	6
stop, no, don't	—	22

Fig. 3. Perceptions and evaluations of alcohol by college drug users (□, total score: 4104) and nonusers (■, total score: 4117).

the dangers of using drugs and alcohol. They view drugs and alcohol in close relationship to dependency and addiction and are much more preoccupied with the possibility of death, that drugs and alcohol kill. Nonusers are strongly negative in their attitudes and evaluations and characterize drinking and taking drugs as stupid and self-destructive. They think of drugs and alcohol in general terms, showing less familiarity with slang terms and paraphernalia.

The frequent users show a tendency to view marijuana, alcohol, and drugs as sources of entertainment and relaxation. They relate drugs more to friends, parties, and social events. In contrast to the nonusers, they do not pay much attention to issues of legality or crime. The users are naturally more familiar with the various types and brands of drugs and alcohol and with their effects in terms of producing altered states of mind. However, they show considerably less concern with loss of control and less awareness of the harmful effects of drug use on health.

The differences between users and nonusers are fairly consistent across the themes (marijuana, drugs) used in the representation of the drug domain and set the two groups apart. As illustrated in the schematic presentation in Fig. 4, these differences (e.g., perceived harm vs enjoyment) offer useful parameters for differentiating nonusers from users along several relevant dimensions of perceptions and evaluations. The differential trends that emerge across the themes can then be used to identify user and nonuser type perceptual and evaluative dispositions in the domains (drugs, family relations) found to be significantly related to drug use.

"Self, Family" Domain

The following themes were used in the representation of self and family: me, I am, family, and father. The users' self image was more narrow and self-centered than the nonusers'. Although both groups of college students expressed basically positive attitudes toward self, the users expressed greater emotional ambivalence and mood swings. The users conveyed greater feelings of depression and dissatisfaction, boredom, and loneliness. Nonusers appeared to be more positive, optimistic, and relaxed about themselves. They demonstrated more goal orientation and stressed their intellectual attributes and identity as students.

The users also expressed more emotional ambivalence in regard to family. They view family with more emphasis on emotional ties and express more concern with family problems, fights, and separation. Non-

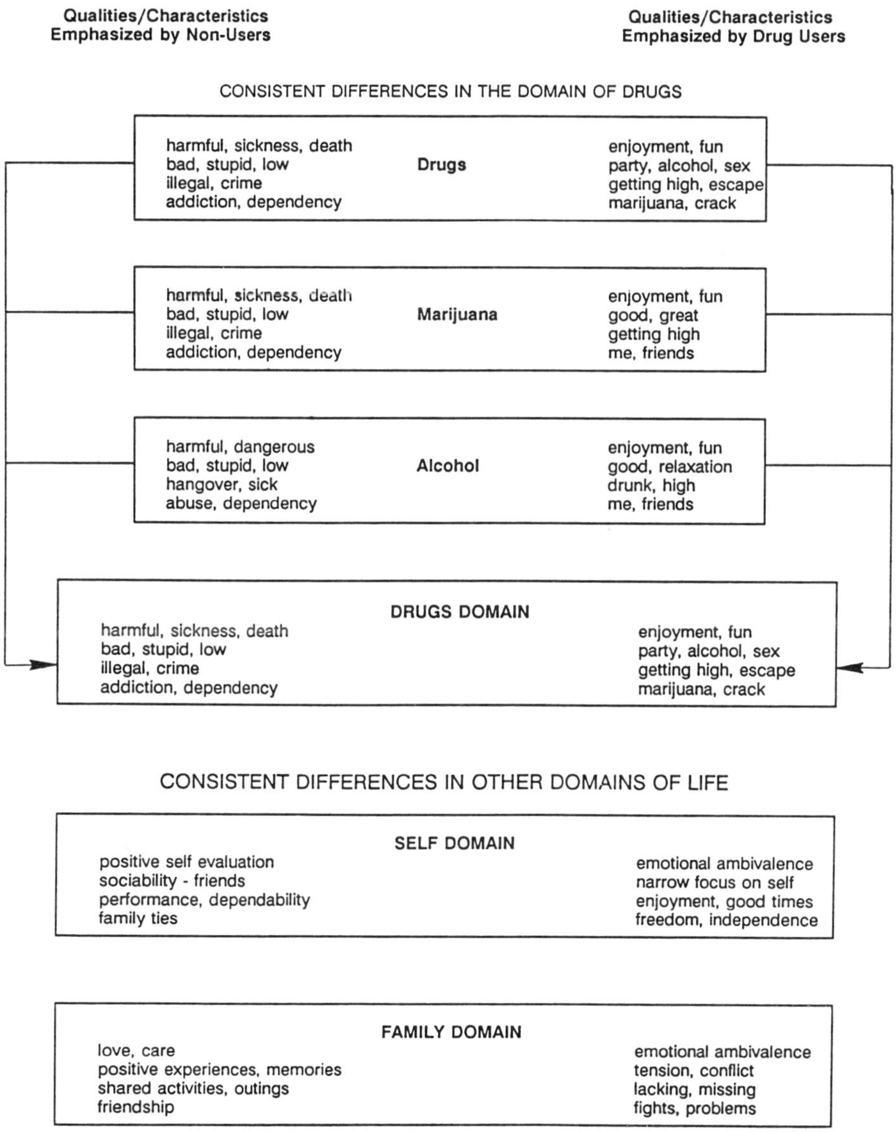

Fig. 4. Perceptions and attitudes differentiating nonusers and drug users.

users think more of good family memories of togetherness and shared experiences and place more weight on the family as a source of happiness and friendship. Differences were particularly noted with regard to perceptions of the father. Users have a more affect-laden image of father, expressing not only great love but also strong feelings of dissatisfaction and alienation. The users were much more explicitly negative in describing father as mean, hateful, and hurting. The nonusers' relationship to father appears to be more positive and harmonious. Nonusers attribute to father more traditional characteristics such as leadership, discipline, and respect.

The comparison of users and nonusers reveals variations in subjective representations that are at the source of different attitudes and behaviors. The findings present new insights into how behavior has its foundation in different representations of reality.

A Multidimensional Assessment of Psychological Dispositions Differentiating Drug Users from Nonusers

The preceding results show that drug users and nonusers differ in perceptions and evaluations and that these differences are not isolated but involve broader trends in subjective representations, reflecting two frames of reference that are internally consistent and empirically identifiable. The following analysis works in the opposite direction. It tests how useful and effective the AGA-based perceptual, representational data is to identify drug users and nonusers.

One way to test this relationship was to examine how effective AGA-based perceptual/evaluative scores calculated on the 400 students individually are to identify who is a user and who is a nonuser. Three main scores were developed to measure the similarities between the individual and the group along three main dimensions of the representational system.

1. Individual perceptual similarity scores indicate the extent to which the responses produced by each subject correspond more closely to the dominant response patterns of drug users or nonusers. In this study the response distributions of comparable, independent samples of 200 frequent users and 200 nonusers provided the reference points.
2. Individual evaluative scores were generated on each of the 24 variables based on the evaluative content of the individual response distributions.
3. Individual dominance scores were based on the number of responses produced to each of the 24 variables by each respondent.

Table 3
Canonical Discriminant Functions

Fcn	Eigenvalue	Pct of Variance	Cum Pct	Canonical Corr	After Fcn	Wilks' Lambda	Chi-square	DF	Sig
1*	.5751	100.00	100.00	.6042	0	.6349	169.679	49	.0000

*marks the 1 canonical discriminant functions remaining in the analysis.

Table 4
Classification Results

Actual group	No. of cases	Predicted group membership 1	2
Group 1 Users	200	161 80.5%	39 19.5%
Group 2 Nonusers	200	52 26.0%	148 74.0%

Percent of "grouped" cases correctly classified: 77.25%

These individual perceptual, evaluative, and dominance score sets calculated on each theme for each student were analyzed to assess their combined effectiveness to identify whether individual students fit more closely into the user group or the nonuser group. Discriminant function analysis was used to calculate the accuracy of identification made on the basis of these scores (Table 3). The classification results presented in Table 4 show a strong correspondence between AGA-based perceptual/attitudinal information and actual behavior: drug user vs nonuser.

Discussion

Differences in Perceptions and Evaluations Indicative of Drug Use

It may be argued that the findings demonstrating that drug users and nonusers perceive drugs differently and that users view drugs more as a source of fun and entertainment whereas nonusers perceive them more as a source of harm confirm essentially common-sense expectations to the point of being trivial. Not only do the findings confirm educated or even trivial expectations, they are also informative on trends of perceptions and evaluations that have not been measured and systematically related to drug use. These trends of the users and nonusers describe two separate systems of subjective representation that serve as the foundation of the observable differences in actual behavior.

Although the present research did not aim to identify perceptual and evaluative differences in all domains that bear on people's choices to use or not to use drugs, the results offer substantial support that drug use and nonuse have their foundation in such representational dispositions or structures that will become more fully accessible in further investigations.

Since the application of the AGA method to the study of subjective systems of representation related to drug use is of relatively recent origin, many of the intriguing questions about personality organization and the organization of systems of representation will require more systematic investigations. Nevertheless, the present findings have sufficiently broad foundation with several practical and theoretical implications.

Users and nonusers differ in their systems of subjective representation along several dimensions related to drug use. Furthermore, these differences in representational structures are empirically identifiable and provide an empirical foundation for a systematic investigation of representational systems and their behavioral implications.

Prevention Evaluation

The results obtained at all three levels of the analysis show that the perceptions of the drug users and nonusers differ widely and consistently. The differences show high internal consistency across themes of the same domain. In the drug domain, for example, drug users viewed marijuana, alcohol, and drugs all as sources of entertainment and relaxation and showed much less awareness of risking loss of control or endangering health, which were the major concerns of the nonusers in all contexts.

As the present findings illustrate, drug users and nonusers differ consistently from each other on a host of psychological dispositions. Second, the results show that these perceptual and evaluative differences set users and nonusers clearly apart. The capability to identify perceptual and evaluative tendencies that differentiate users and nonusers opens up interesting new opportunities to examine individual people or groups with regard to their internal psychological dispositions related to drug use. The analytic capability demonstrated here suggests several promising applications.

First, it opens new vistas for our interest in identifying latent dispositions—vulnerabilities, psychological sensitivities in terms of prevention and evaluation that are likely to lead to drug use.

Second, the analytic capabilities available for such assessment suggest practical ways for measuring the psychological effects of prevention programs designed to reduce vulnerabilities and strengthen psychological dispositions that will reduce the tendency to engage in drug use.

Third, these new analytic capabilities promise new opportunities to evaluate the effects of various prevention programs with regard to their effectiveness to move people from views and evaluations characteristic of habitual drug users toward perceptions and attitudes characteristic of nonusers. Since the changes measured involve changes in psychological dispositions related to drug use, the research strategy offers a new capability to evaluate highly diverse programs with regard to their relative effectiveness to achieve internal changes related to drug use.

Mapping Subjective Representations: Their Use in Predicting Behavior

The analytic method demonstrates that users and nonusers differ along a set of perceptions and evaluations. The findings offer strong empirical support to the representational theory of behavioral organization. The results of the discriminant function analysis show that differences identified in subjective images and meanings can be used with a high degree of accuracy to identify people who are users and nonusers. In testing this relationship between systems of representations and behavior, the results of the discriminant function analysis have offered substantive evidence that systems of subjective representations play an intensive role in shaping behavior, at least, in the context of drug use. Since this relationship between subjective representations and behavior is likely to vary in the context of behaviors other than drug use, this relationship naturally requires broader examination. Data are being presently examined in the field of alcohol and tobacco dependency and systems of subjective representation.

In view of the advanced medical knowledge accumulating on neuropharmacological dimensions of drug use, the present findings on the perceptual/representational correlates of drug use suggest new ways to attack the complex and evasive psychological variables more systematically.

The findings empirically support the viability of a research strategy that may have appeared overly ambitious at first sight. They indicate that it is possible to identify and analyze perceptual/representational dispositions, that is, internal states responsible for differences in behavior—drug use, nonuse—including eventually internal states of certain transitional stages. A simple logical extension of this capability could allow for several practical applications presently needed. It could provide an empirical assessment of vulnerabilities and resistance characteristic of various populations that appear to be at high risk based on available statistics and epidemiological indicators. It could also be used in the evaluation of prevention and treatment programs with regard to their psychological effects on changing perceptions and systems of representation, along the criteria associated with stable drug-free states.

In general, this research strategy provides new opportunities to expand our knowledge of internal states associated with drug use and to gain insights into certain critical psychological variables affecting drug use, variables mostly beyond the reach of empirical assessment.

Acknowledgments

The research reported here was sponsored by the Department of Education and FIPSE, the Fund for the Improvement of Post-Secondary Education. The views expressed here are those of the authors.

References

[1]R. J. Craig (1986) *The Personality Structure of Heroin Addicts* (Research monograph no. 74). National Institute of Drug Abuse, US Government Printing Office, Washington, DC, pp. 25–36.

[2]A. R. Zeiner, T. Stanitis, M. Spurgeon, and N. Nichols (1985) Treatment of alcoholism and concomitant drugs of abuse. *Alcohol* **2,** 555–559.

[3]G. Krampen and A. Von Eye (1984) Generalized expectancies of drug delinquents, other delinquents, and a control sample. *Addict. Behav.* **9,** 421–423.

[4]A. P. Jurich and C. J. Polson (1984) Reasons for drug use: Comparison of drug users and abusers. *Psychol. Rep.* **55,** 371–378.

[5]A. Weidman (1983) The compulsive adolescent substance abuser: Psychological differentiation and family process. *J. Drug Education* **13,** 161–172.

[6]B. Segal and P. F. Merenda (1975) Locus of control, sensation seeking, and

drug and alcohol use in college students. *Drug Forum* **4,** 349–369.

[7]O. Doherty and G. Matthews (1988) Personality characteristics of opiate addicts. *Pers. Individual Differences* **9,** 171–172.

[8]T. E. Dielman, P. C. Campanelli, J. T. Shope, and A. T. Butchart (1987) Susceptibility to peer pressure, self esteem, and health locus of control as correlates of adolescent substance abuse. *Health Education Q.* **14,** 207–221.

[9]D. C. Des Jarlais (1986) *Locus of Control and Need for Control Among Heroin Users* (NIDA Research Monograph 74). National Institute of Drug Abuse, US Government Printing Office, Washington, DC, pp. 37–44.

[10]A. L. Olton (1985) The effect of locus of control and perceptions of school environment on outcome in three school drug abuse prevention programs. *J. Drug Education* **15,** 157–169.

[11]J. H. Malvin, J. M. Moskowitz, E. Schaps, and G. A. Schaeffer (1985) Evaluation of two school based alternative programs. *J. Alcohol Drug Education* **30,** 98–108.

[12]D. J. Rohsenow, R. E. Smith, and S. Johnson (1985) Stress management training as a prevention program for heavy social drinkers. *Addict. Behav.* **10,** 45–54.

[13]S. J. Biggs, M. P. Bender, and J. Foreman (1983) Are there psychological differences between persistent solvent abusing delinquents and delinquents who do not use solvents? *J. Adolescence* **6,** 71–86.

[14]K. J. McBride (1982) I-E scores of drug abusing offenders: The influence of social desirability. *Criminal Justice Behav.* **9,** 177–183.

[15]P. B. Sutker and A. N. Allian (1988) Issues in personality conceptualizations of addictive behaviors. *J. Consult. Clin. Psychol.* **56,** 172–182.

[16]R. J. Craig (1988) Psychological functioning of cocaine free basers and derived from objective psychological tests. *J. Clin. Psychol.* **44,** 599–606.

[17]A. Burr (1984) The ideologies of despair: A symbolic interpretation of punks and skinheads usage of barbiturates. *Soc. Sci. Med.* **19,** 929–938.

[18]K. B. Stein, W. F. Soskin, and S. J. Korchin (1975) Drug use among disaffected high school youth. *J. Drug Education* **5,** 193–203.

[19]A. M. Nicholi (1974) Emotional determinants of LSD ingestion. *J. Am. Coll. Health Assoc.* **22,** 223–225.

[20]R. E. Horman (1973) Alienation and student drug use. *Int. J. Addict.* **8,** 325–331.

[21]R. D. Hays, A. W. Stacy, K. F. Widaman, and M. R. DiMatteo (1986) Multistage path models of adolescent alcohol and drug use: A reanalysis. *J. Drug Issues* **16,** 357–369.

[22]B. A. Rouse and J. A. Ewing (1974) Student drug use, risk taking, and alienation. *J. Am. Coll. Health Assoc.* **22,** 226–230.

[23]R. T. Dull (1983) An empirical examination of the anomie theory of drug use. *J. Drug Education* **13,** 49–62.

[24]R. A. Steffenhagen, J. M. Polich, and S. Lash (1978) Alienation, delinquency, and patterns of drug use. *Int. J. Social Psychiatry* **24,** 125–137.

[25]J. D. Hundleby (1986) Personality and the prediction of delinquency and drug use: A follow up study of school boys. *Br. J. Criminology* **26,** 129–146.

[26]H. C. Triandis and V. Vassiliou (1967) *Componential Analysis of Subjective Culture.* University of Illinois, Urbana, IL.

[27]E. C. Tolman (1948) Cognitive maps in rats and men. *Psychol. Rev.* **55,** 189–208.

[28]R. M. Downs and D. Stea (1973) *Image and Environment: Cognitive Mapping and Spacial Behavior.* Aldine, Chicago, IL.

[29]M. I. Posner and S. W. Keele (1968) On the genesis of abstract ideas. *J. Exp. Psychol.* **77,** 353–363.

[30]R. M. Shepard and S. Chipman (1970) Second order isomorphism of internal representations: Shapes of state. *Cognitive Psychol.* **1,** 1–7.

[31]G. A. Miller (1967) Psycholinguistic approaches to the study of communication, in *Journeys in Science.* D. Arm, ed. University of New Mexico Press, Albuquerque, NM.

[32]C. E. Osgood, G. J. Suci, and P. H. Tannenbaum (1957) *The Measurement of Meaning.* University of Illinois Press, Urbana, IL.

[33]B. Whorf (1957) *Language, Thought and Reality.* Technological Press/Wiley, New York.

[34]C. Noble (1952) An analysis of meaning. *Psychol. Rev.* **54,** 421–440.

[35]J. Deese (1965) *The Structure of Associations In Language and Thought.* John Hopkins University Press, Baltimore, MD.

[36]L. B. Szalay and J. Deese (1978) *Subjective Meaning and Culture: An Assessment Through Word Associations.* Lawrence Erlbaum/Wiley, Hillsdale, NJ.

[37]L. B. Szalay, W. T. Moon, D. A. Lysne, and J. A. Bryson (1971) *A Lexicon of Selected U.S.–Korean Communication Themes.* Center for Research in Social Systems, American Institutes for Research, Kensington, MD.

[38]L. B. Szalay and J. A. Bryson (1973) Measurement of psychocultural distance: A comparison of American Blacks and Whites. *J. Pers. Soc. Psychol.* **26,** 166–177.

[39]L. B. Szalay, C. Windle, and D. A. Lysne (1970) Attitude measurement by free verbal associations. *J. Soc. Psychol.* **82,** 43–55.

Treatment of Nicotine Dependence in Substance Use Disorder Patients

Anne M. Joseph

Introduction

Smoking is responsible for over 400,000 deaths each year in the United States, more than three times the number of deaths annually resulting from alcohol and 100 times the deaths resulting from cocaine.[1] Our culture draws many distinctions between addiction to tobacco and alcohol and other drugs, however. The drug dependency treatment field has traditionally regarded tobacco use as less dangerous than alcohol or other drug use. In part, this is because of fear of jeopardizing the success of drug dependency treatment by treating nicotine dependence, and many staff are themselves nicotine dependent.

Recognition of the high prevalence of nicotine addiction in patients with other substance use disorders has stimulated interest in the challenge of treating nicotine addiction in patients with alcohol and drug problems, and several national developments have led the drug and alcohol treatment community to reconsider the usual approach to smoking. The physically addicting properties of nicotine have been recognized by the American Psychiatric Association through establishing diagnostic categories of nicotine dependence and nicotine withdrawal in 1980.[2] The Surgeon General's Report on Nicotine Addiction and investigation of the role of nicotine replacement therapy in smoking cessation have empha-

From: *Drug and Alcohol Abuse Reviews, Vol. 4: Drug Abuse Treatment*
Ed: R. R. Watson ©1992 The Humana Press Inc.

sized the physiological aspects of nicotine use.[3,4] Recognition of the dangers associated with environmental tobacco smoke and the nonsmokers' rights movement have led to further restrictions on smoking in public buildings, including medical institutions. Controversy about the appropriate management of substance use disorder patients in the setting of smoke-free hospitals abounds.

This chapter reviews the relationship between tobacco and other substance use, compares patterns of substance use, and describes the consequences of tobacco use in substance disorder populations. Available scientific data on management of nicotine dependence in patients with other substance use disorders and controversies in the field is also discussed. Preliminary investigation in this area has yielded most information about alcoholic populations; data from patients with other drug dependency problems are referenced when available.

Prevalence

General Population

There is a consistent association between cigaret consumption and alcohol use in representative samples of the general population. Klatsky et al. found that heavy drinkers among a large sample of Black, White, or Oriental adults of both sexes ($n = 91{,}659$) were two to three times more likely than nondrinkers to be cigaret smokers.[5] Friedman and coworkers found that a greater percentage of smokers than nonsmokers fell in the heaviest drinking categories (25 vs 9% for men).[6] Studies in other Western developed countries confirm a moderately strong relationship in the general population between tobacco and alcohol consumption of similar magnitude in both sexes.[7,8]

Alcoholic Populations

Evidence suggests that virtually all alcoholic patients of both sexes are cigaret smokers. Over 90% of alcoholic male and female outpatients in Canada were cigaret smokers, far more than in the general population.[9] Ashley et al. reported that among 582 male and 83 female alcoholic inpatients, 92% of men and 95% of females were current smokers.[10] Data from Walton and Ayers et al. confirm the high rates of smoking among alcoholics.[11,12]

The prevalence of smoking in the general population has declined remarkably in the last decade, especially among White males in higher socioeconomic groups.[13] In 1965, 60% of the general male population smoked cigarets, compared to 42% in 1980, whereas in 1965, 90% of alcoholic males smoked compared with 86% in 1979.[14] The minimal decline in smoking prevalence among alcoholic populations may reflect factors known to be associated with difficulty quitting, such as lower socioeconomic status and educational level, or there may be an interaction with other substance use disorders.

Patterns of Smoking Among Alcoholic Users

It is suggested that addictive behaviors are powerful cues for one another. Drinkers smoke more heavily when consuming alcohol.[15] Griffiths et al. studied alcoholic subjects under controlled and blinded conditions, and found that ethanol induced smoking independent of the social situation or schedule of availability of alcohol.[16] Cigarets are puffed more intensively when used in combination with alcohol.[17] This raises the possibility that abstinence from alcohol may be associated with a decrease in tobacco consumption.

There is a moderately strong relationship between *heavy* drinking and *heavy* smoking. Craig and Van Netta reported 31% and 27% of male and female heavy drinkers (≥7 drinks/d) smoked >1 pack of cigarets/d, whereas corresponding percentages among male and female nondrinkers were 13% and 7%.[18] Some 24% of alcoholic men and 37% of alcoholic women were heavy smokers (>40 cigarets/d), compared to 2.5% and 0.9%, respectively in the general population in Canada.[9] This relationship appears consistent across nationality and gender, as well as in adolescent and adult populations.[7]

Burling et al. found that smokers who avoided alcohol were more successful in reducing their levels of smoking than those who did not.[19] For an individual who drinks moderately, but has stopped smoking, alcohol has been found to be associated with from one-fifth to one-half of smoking relapse episodes.[20]

Smoking Patterns and Other Drug Use in Patients

Some 97% of opiate addicts in treatment were reported to use cigarets daily,[21] but there is little other data available on the relationship between tobacco use in patients with other drug use problems. Patterns of initiating use of alcohol, drugs, and tobacco have been studied looking for common etiologies to addictive disorders. Data suggest adolescents start using beer and wine, and then progress to tobacco and hard liquor, and that marijuana is seldom used without first using tobacco.[8,21] It is possible that prevention of tobacco use may have an effect on future illicit drug use, although this has never been proven.

Significance

The serious medical consequences of smoking will not be reviewed in detail, but tobacco is responsible for 85% of lung cancer deaths, 90% of chronic obstructive lung disease cases, and 35% of cardiovascular disease deaths in the United States.[1] Tobacco and alcohol act as synergistic risk factors in several common conditions. The odds of a heavy smoker and heavy drinker developing esophageal cancer is 156 times that of a nondrinker, nonsmoker.[22] Smoking cessation is associated with a decrease in the relative risk for esophageal cancer.[23] It is established that laryngeal[24,25] and oropharyngeal tumors[26] occur more commonly in smokers who also drink alcohol. Use of both substances increases the risk of stomach cancer,[27] tuberculosis,[28] toxic amblyopia,[11] and duodenal ulcer.[29]

Patients who undergo structured substance use disorder treatment are usually young and have not yet developed irreversible medical consequences of smoking. Therefore, this is an ideal target population for prevention of physical complications from smoking and drinking. The most important modifiable risk factor affecting future health for patients who are recovering from alcohol and drug addiction is tobacco use.

Comparisons Between Alcohol and Tobacco Use

It is useful to recognize similarities between patterns of alcohol and tobacco use, though there are many important differences. Inhaled nicotine reaches the brain 7 s after inhalation and has an extremely short half-life (90–120 min). Smokers can precisely regulate nicotine dosing through both frequency and depth of inhalation. Alcohol takes longer to affect behavior and has more lasting effects. Overuse of alcohol is associated with more legal and social problems because nicotine does not impair performance.

Approximately 90% of smokers are physically dependent on nicotine.[3] Even smokers who use only a few cigarets per day are likely to become physically dependent, and do so over a relatively short period of time (often within a year).[30] In contrast, 80–90% or more of alcohol consumers are occasional users and not "addicted."[31] Because our culture is becoming less tolerant of smoking, it is likely that in the future nicotine use will play a role in employability and personal relationships, but to date, the commonly recognized consequences of nicotine addiction are medical and personal. There are more data to support the goal of reduced consumption for alcohol-dependent patients than nicotine-dependent patients, for whom abstinence is usually the only successful treatment method.[30]

The recovery process for both nicotine and alcohol dependence is most commonly self-directed, and accomplished without formal or structured treatment. In both cases, those who do recover without formal help have fewer problems than those who require treatment. Both substances are heavily advertised, legal, and easily available. They contribute significantly to the national economy and federal and state tax revenue; treatment therefore must address advertising and economic aspects of substance use. Relapse rates for treatment of a variety of substance use disorders, including alcohol, tobacco, and heroin, are remarkably similar.[32] Similar factors are reported to precipitate relapse to nicotine and alcohol use, including stress, conflict, and social pressure.

Interest in Quitting

Many professionals feel futile giving smoking cessation advice to drug and alcohol treatment patients, citing a "lack of interest" in quitting as a certain predictor of failure. Data from several investigators suggest patients under treatment for alcohol problems may be more open to consider smoking cessation than anticipated.

We studied 912 consecutive patients admitted for inpatient treatment of substance use at the Minneapolis VA Medical Center. In all, 77% of patients were current cigaret smokers, and 80% smoked >1 pack/d. A hospital-wide policy was implemented in 1988 that completely banned smoking in the medical center, including psychiatry and drug dependency wards. The drug treatment program introduced an intervention to address nicotine dependence in the inpatient program at the same time. We compared responses to a standardized questionnaire about smoking habits and attitudes toward smoking cessation in a group of chemically

Table 1
Results of Prepolicy and Postpolicy Intervention Survey

	Prepolicy	Postpolicy	P
Admission questionnaire	n = 407	n - 299	
Cigaret smokers, %	77	76	.91
Current smokers	n = 312	n = 226	
Want to quit, %	36	62	<.001
Interest in quitting in hospital, %	24	61	<.001
Discharge questionnaire	n = 336	n = 252	
Cigaret smokers, %	75	78	.99
Current smokers	n = 252	n = 197	
Abstain from smoking >1 wk, %	9	41	<.001
Cut down in hospital, %	46	93	<.001
Not smoking regularly, %	19	58	<.001
Feel quit threatens sobriety, %	28	32	.22
No plan to change smoking habits, %	12	6	<.001

dependent patients admitted for inpatient treatment before and after the policy was implemented.

In all, 36% of patients in the prepolicy group said they wanted to quit smoking, compared to 62% in the postpolicy group ($p < .001$). Moreover, 24% said they were interested in quitting during the hospitalization before the policy, compared to 61% after the policy ($p < .001$). Rates of early termination of treatment did not change, and 41% of patients hospitalized in the postpolicy group abstained from smoking for more than 1 wk during hospitalization *(see* Table 1). We concluded that concurrent intervention for nicotine addiction during inpatient treatment is feasible, and associated with a temporary reduction in smoking and increased motivation to quit smoking.[33]

Koslowski et al. interviewed 289 consecutive clients in Canada interested in drug or alcohol treatment. Among 86% who were current smokers 53% said they "moderately" or "very much" wanted to give up smoking, and 46% said they were interested in a smoking treatment program. Another questionnaire administered to 122 consecutive patients indicated that 78% wanted treatment for their drug or alcohol problem *prior* to receiving treatment for smoking. Some 31% were "moderately" to "very interested" in receiving treatment at the same time.[34] In another series of

805 alcohol and drug users, 25% said they were willing to try to quit smoking at the same time as their other treatment.[30] These data suggest that a significant proportion of substance use disorder patients are interested in treatment for nicotine dependence at the same time or after treatment for other substance use.

Approximately 1000 patients were asked about the difficulty of quitting use of the substance for which they were seeking treatment relative to the difficulty in quitting cigarets. In all, 57% said that cigarets would be harder to stop than their problem substance, despite the fact that cigarets were generally rated as less pleasurable than alcohol or drugs. Alcohol-dependent persons were four times more likely than drug-dependent persons to say their strongest urges for cigarets were at least as great as their strongest urges for their problem substance.[35]

Experience in Quitting

Alcohol Users in the General Population

Zimmerman et al. examined the relationship between alcohol use and smoking cessation in a sample of 2115 adults in the general population. He found that heavy drinkers were less likely to try to stop smoking, but quitting drinking was strongly related to success at smoking cessation, given an attempt to stop smoking. Quitting drinking, however, was overall associated with fewer attempts to quit smoking than continued drinking.[36]

Substance-Dependent Populations

Bobo et al. interviewed a group of 73 recovering alcoholics and found 19% had stopped smoking, a mean of 36.2 mo following treatment. Markers of successful smoking cessation were:

1. Less severe substance abuse history;
2. Fewer chemical dependency admissions;
3. Briefer alcohol abuse history;
4. Lower MAST subscale scores;
5. Fewer smoking-related problems; and
6. Lighter smoking rates during chemical dependency treatment.

Of those successful at stopping smoking, 93% reported uninterrupted sobriety since discharge. The data suggest that individuals with more severe substance abuse histories may be less successful quitting cigarets.[37]

Another series of questions addressed the concern that the additional stress of smoking cessation would endanger recovery from alcoholism. The respondents disagreed with the statements, "Sometimes the stress of trying to avoid cigarettes has caused me to drink alcohol," and "When I first quit smoking, I really wanted to drink again." Based on their experience, this small group of patients recommended smoking cessation after completion of treatment.[38]

In a study of male and female alcohol abusers, Miller et al. observed that relapse to smoking by a pretreatment nonsmoker was associated with continued alcohol use. Smoking cessation by pretreatment smokers was associated with successful control of drinking, though pretreatment nonsmoking was not. This raises the possibility that smoking cessation might improve alcohol treatment outcomes.[39]

The association observed between smoking and alcohol use has led to speculation that abstinence from alcohol might be accompanied by a compensatory increase in smoking, but a relevant study suggests the contrary. Maletzky et al. interviewed alcoholic patients upon entering treatment and several weeks after completion of treatment. All patients in the alcoholic sample were smokers ($n = 57$). Those alcoholics who were abstinent following treatment smoked slightly fewer cigarets per day than those who did not succeed in treatment.[40] These studies suggest alcoholics with a less severe history, are more likely to attempt and succeed at smoking cessation, but the data are very limited and do not confirm how many recovering alcoholics attempt cessation.

Nicotine Dependency Treatment for Substance Abuse Patients

Pros and Cons

Substance use treatment lore holds that alcohol and drug addiction is a more disruptive and less socially acceptable process than tobacco dependence, and that smoking cessation would be stressful and might threaten the attainment and maintenance of sobriety. The assumption that smoking interventions will harm outcomes of chemical dependency treatment is not based on scientific data, however.

It was once considered essential to treat patients with multiple addictions (e.g., drugs and alcohol) sequentially, but combined treatment is now the norm, exploiting the common themes in treatment. Some professionals believe that addressing nicotine addiction at the same time as other substances will enhance the treatment process, because certain cues may be associated with the act of substance consumption. It is possible that trying to stop drinking, for example, while maintaining smoking is more difficult than stopping use of both substances at the same time. Simultaneous treatment might also demonstrate a more consistent approach to addictions.

The 1987 Surgeon General's Report demonstrates that tobacco does meet standard definitions of drug addiction:

1. The user's behavior is largely controlled by a psychoactive substance and the drug is reinforcing;
2. Continued use is accompanied by tolerance;
3. Physical dependence occurs;
4. There is a characteristic withdrawal syndrome; and
5. There is a tendency after abstinence to relapse.[3]

Effects of Smoking Cessation on Substance Abuse Disorder Treatment

To address the concern that including nicotine in drug dependency treatment would harm treatment outcomes, we conducted structured interviews with two groups of patients about smoking, alcohol, and drug use behavior approx 1 yr after completion of inpatient treatment. One group was hospitalized in a "traditional" program that only discouraged smoking. The second group was hospitalized after June 1988, when a hospital policy banning smoking and a structured smoking cessation program designed for use in the inpatient drug dependency treatment program were introduced. All patients in the second group agreed to treatment for nicotine dependency upon admission. The program included didactic sessions on physical and psychological dependence on nicotine, consequences of smoking, films, and group sessions.

Descriptive data from patients admitted prior to program implementation were similar to data from patients admitted after the change in policy. Alcohol was the drug of choice for 72%, cocaine the drug of choice for 15%, and 70% used more than one substance. Some 79% of patients were cigaret smokers at the time of admission. Prepolicy patients (n = 156) were interviewed a mean of 16.2 mo after discharge from the hospital, and postpolicy patients (n = 163) were interviewed a mean of 10.7 mo after discharge.

"Improvement" in chemical dependency, defined as less or no substance abuse (excluding nicotine), was reported by 97% of prepolicy patients, compared to 89% of postpolicy patients (difference not statistically significant). A conservative assumption that all study nonrespondents were chemical dependency and smoking treatment failures did not result in significant differences in treatment outcomes pre- and postpolicy. At the time of followup, 21% of prepolicy patients smoked less than they had on admission, compared to 19% of postpolicy patients (difference not statistically significant).

In all, 13 postpolicy patients quit smoking, compared to 5 prepolicy patients ($p < .05$). Narrative comments indicated that most postpolicy patients found the hospital smoking ban acceptable, but many resented the mandatory nature of the cessation program. Many patients noted difficulty attending aftercare meetings outside the hospital setting, where there was limited support for smoking cessation and smoking was ubiquitous.

Although this study was limited by the use of historical controls and self-reported drug, alcohol, and tobacco use data, we concluded that a smoke-free inpatient drug treatment program was associated with a slightly higher rate of smoking cessation without a significant decrease in drug and alcohol treatment outcomes, although there was a trend in this direction.[41]

Staff Attitudes

Many treatment programs have staff members who are recovering from addiction disorders, and many are smokers. This is postulated to explain reluctance on the part of treatment professionals to address the issue of tobacco dependence. Investigators in the field report ongoing controversy among administrators and staff in treatment centers about smoking policy, and practical and moral issues concerning treatment of nicotine dependence.

Bobo and Gilchrist examined attitudes among staff in chemical dependency treatment centers toward smoking cessation. A total of 311 professionals from 23 treatment centers were asked about the prevalence of smoking, timing, and advisability of interventions for smoking. Some 35% of staff were regular smokers. Smoking staff were significantly less likely to urge cessation, and 53% thought 1 yr of alcohol abstinence was an appropriate point for smoking intervention, though only 33% actually did so. In all, 46% thought alcoholic patients would have more difficulty quitting cigarets than nonalcoholic patients.[42]

A survey of administrators of all the chemical dependency facilities ($n = 227$) in Minnesota in 1988 was conducted to determine attitudes about tobacco use in chemical dependency treatment facilities and the effect of an educational intervention on chemical dependency treatment facilities' smoking policies. Although many administrators agreed that nicotine dependence should be treated like other drug dependencies, a minority of facilities included tobacco treatment in their program. Frequently cited barriers to creating a smoke-free facility included fear of losing patients and staff smoking habits. Many directors supported legislation mandating smoke-free treatment facilities.[43]

Controversies in Treatment

A few of the programs that do treat nicotine addiction based on the "Minnesota Model" regard complete abstinence as the only goal of treatment. This generally precludes use of nicotine replacement therapy, a treatment that has been shown in randomized, double-blind, placebo-controlled trials to augment quit rates, particularly among heavy smokers who are physically dependent on nicotine.[3] These programs teach patients to use the same tools that are effective in the management of withdrawal and craving symptoms experienced with other substances.

It is well known that symptoms of acute nicotine withdrawal include anxiety, difficulty concentrating, and sleep disturbance. Physical symptoms of withdrawal from nicotine peak in 48–72 h and are complete in 10–12 d.[4] Although this uncomfortable period may be best passed with the structure and support of the inpatient setting, some professionals have been reluctant to subject patients to this syndrome during treatment. They recommend that patients address smoking after a period of abstinence from drugs and alcohol, although this approach has never been formally tested.

Other unanswered questions in this setting include the need for staff to be tobacco-free and appropriate management of tobacco use during treatment. Use of drugs or alcohol during treatment usually meets serious consequences. Many professionals fear that equal treatment for smoking during treatment will discourage program participation. Smokers are rarely able to quit on their first try, however, so slip-ups should be anticipated, particularly in this population where smoking cessation may not be a priority. Strategies to educate patients about nicotine addiction in such treatment settings have been described.[44]

Smokers' rights groups compare the current nonsmokers' rights movement to the Prohibition drive.[45] Analogies are limited, however, because the former is more scientifically based; all levels of tobacco consumption have proven dangerous, and there are established risks associated with passive smoking. Nevertheless, our society is not tolerant of moralistic overtones in admonishing smoking behavior, and this approach may promote resistance to educational efforts. It is likely that it will be necessary to acknowledge distinctions between drug and alcohol and nicotine addiction for some time to come. Rather than assume that recovering alcoholic and drug-dependent patients need protection from nicotine dependency treatment, we must begin to investigate the most effective approach to this common problem thoughtfully.

Randomized trials are needed to determine the most effective timing for nicotine dependency interventions, the utility of nicotine replacement therapy, and the effect of including nicotine dependency treatment in program participation rates, a fundamental concern. As long as the substance abuse treatment field denies the problem of nicotine addiction, results from the best work in the field will be subject to medical failure through premature cardiac and pulmonary disease.

References

[1]US Department of Health and Human Services (1990) *The Health Benefits of Smoking Cessation.* US Department of Health and Human Services, Public Health Service, Centers for Disease Control, Center for Chronic Disease Prevention and Health Promotion, Office on Smoking and Health. DHHS Publication No. (CDC) 90-8416.

[2]American Psychiatric Association (1987) *Diagnostic and Statistical Manual of Mental Disorders*, 3rd ed., rev. American Psychiatric Association, Washington, DC.

[3]US Department of Health and Human Services (1988) *The Health Consequences of Smoking: Nicotine Addiction.* US Department of Health and Human Services, Public Health Service, Centers for Disease Control, Center for Chronic Disease Prevention and Health Promotion, Office on Smoking and Health, Rockville, MD.

[4]N. L. Benowitz (1988) Pharmacologic aspects of cigarette smoking and

nicotine addiction. *N. Engl. J. Med.* **319,** 1318-1330.

[5]A. L. Klatsky, G. D. Friedman, A. B. Siegelaub, and M. J. Gerard (1977) Alcohol consumption among white, black, or Oriental men and women: Kaiser-Permanente multiphasic health examination data. *Am. J. Epidemiol.* **105,** 311–323.

[6]G. D. Friedman, A. B. Siegelaub, and C. C. Seltzer (1974) Cigarettes, alcohol, coffee and peptic ulcer. *N. Engl. J. Med.* **290,** 469–473.

[7]J. Istvan and J. D. Matarazzo (1984) Tobacco, alcohol, and caffeine use: a review of their interrelationships. *Psychol. Bull.* **95,** 301–326.

[8]K. L. Soeken and R. B. Bausell (1989) Alcohol use and its relationship to other addictive and preventive behaviors. *Addict. Behav.* **14,** 459–464.

[9]K. F. Dreher and J. G. Fraser (1967) Smoking habits of alcoholic out-patients. *Int. J. Addict.* **2,** 259–270.

[10]M. J. Ashley, J. S. Olin, W. H. le Riche, A. Kornaczewski, W. Schmidt, and J. G. Rankin (1981) Morbidity patterns in hazardous drinkers: relevance of demographic, sociologic, drinking and drug use characteristics. *Int. J. Addict.* **16,** 593–625.

[11]R. G. Walton (1972) Smoking and alcoholism: a brief report. *Am. J. Psychiatry* **128,** 1455,1456.

[12]J. Ayers, C. F. Rugg, and D. I. Templer (1976) Alcoholism, cigarette smoking, coffee drinking and extraversion. *J. Stud. Alcohol* **37,** 983–985.

[13]E. J. Hatziandreu, J. P. Pierce, M. Lefkopoulou, M. C. Fiore, S. L. Mills, T. E. Novotny, G. A. Giovino, and R. M. Davis (1990) Quitting smoking in the United States in 1986. *J. Natl. Cancer Inst.* **82,** 1402–1406.

[14]L. T. Koslowski, L. C. Jelinek, and M. A. Pope (1986) Cigarette smoking among alcohol abusers: a continuing and neglected problem. *Can. J. Public Health* **77,** 205–207.

[15]J. E. Henninfield, L. D. Chait, and R. R. Griffiths (1984) Effects of ethanol on cigarette smoking by volunteers without histories of alcoholism. *Psychopharmacology* **82,** 1–5.

[16]R. R. Griffiths, G. E. Bigelow, I. Liebson (1976) Facilitation of human tobacco self-administration by ethanol: a behavioral analysis. *J. Exp. Anal. Behav.* **25,** 279–292.

[17]R. Nil, R. Buzzi, and K. Battig (1984) Effects of single doses of alcohol and caffeine on cigarette smoke puffing behavior. *Pharmacol. Biochem. Behav.* **20,** 583–590.

[18]T. J. Craig and P. A. Van Netta (1977) The association of smoking and drinking habits in a community sample. *J. Stud. Alcohol* **38,** 1434–1439.

[19]T. A. Burling, M. L. Stitzer, G. E. Bigelow, and N. W. Russ (1982) Techniques used by smokers during contingency motivated smoking reduction. *Addict. Behav.* **7,** 397–401.

[20]T. H. Brandon, S. T. Taffany, and T. B. Baker (1986) The process of smoking

relapse, in *Relapse and Recovery in Drug Abuse.* (NIDA Research Monograph No. 72). F. Tims and C. Leukefeld, eds. 104–117, Rockville, MD, National Institute on Drug Abuse.

[21]R. J. Battjes (1988) Smoking as an issue in alcohol and drug abuse treatment. *Addict. Behav.* **13,** 225–230.

[22]N. E. Day and N. Munoz (1982) Cancer of the esophagus, in *Cancer Epidemiology and Prevention.* D. Schottenfeld and J. F. Fraumen, eds. Saunders, Philadelphia, pp. 596–623.

[23]R. Doll and R. Peto (1976) Mortality in relation to smoking: 20 years' observations on male British doctors. *BMJ* **2,** 1525–1536.

[24]D. Burch, G. R. Howe, A. B. Miller, and R. Semenciw (1981) Tobacco, alcohol, asbestos, and nickel in the etiology of cancer of the larynx: a case-control study. *J. Natl. Cancer Inst.* **67,** 1219–1224.

[25]A. J. McMichael (1978) Increases in laryngeal cancer in Britain and Australia in relation to alcohol and tobacco consumption trends. *Lancet* **i,** 1244–1246.

[26]K. Rothman and A. Keller (1972) The effect of joint exposure to alcohol and tobacco on risk of cancer of the mouth and pharynx. *J. Chron. Dis.* **25,** 711–716.

[27]J. Hoey, C. Montvernay, and R. Lambert (1981) Wine and tobacco: risk factors for gastric cancer in France. *Am. J. Epidemiol.* **113,** 668–674.

[28]J. G. Lewis and D. A. Chamberlain (1963) Alcohol consumption and smoking habits in male patients with pulmonary tuberculosis. *Br. J. Prev. Soc. Med.* **17,** 149–152.

[29]S. Sontag, D. Y. Graham, A. Belsito, J. Weiss, A. Farley, R. Grunt, N. Cohen, D. Kinnear, W. Davis, and A. Archambault et al. (1984) Cimetidine, cigarette smoking, and recurrence of duodenal ulcer. *N. Engl. J. Med.* **311,** 689.

[30]L. C. Sobell, M. B. Sobell, L. T. Koslowski, and T. Toneatto (1990) Alcohol or tobacco research versus alcohol and tobacco research. *Br. J. Addict.* **85,** 263–269.

[31]O. F. Pomerleau (1990) What does research on nicotine and tobacco use have to offer alcohol researchers? *Br. J. Addict.* **85,** 247–250.

[32]W. A. Hunt, L. W. Barnett, and L. G. Branch (1971) Relapse rates in addiction programs. *J. Clin. Psychol.* **27,** 455,456.

[33]A. M. Joseph, K. L. Nichol, M. L. Willenbring, J. E. Korn, and L. S. Lysaght (1990) Beneficial effects of treatment of nicotine dependence during an inpatient substance abuse treatment program. *JAMA* **263,** 3043–3046.

[34]L. T. Koslowski, W. Skinner, C. Kent, and M. A. Pope (1989) Prospects for smoking treatment in individuals seeking treatment for alcohol and other drug problems. *Addict. Behav.* **14,** 273–278.

[35]L. T. Koslowski, A. Wilkinson, W. Skinner, C. Kent, T. Franklin, and M. Pope (1989) Comparing tobacco cigarette dependence with other drug dependencies. *JAMA* **261,** 898–901.

[36]R. S. Zimmerman, G. J. Warheit, P. M. Ulbrich, and J. B. Auth (1990) The relationship between alcohol use and attempts and success at smoking cessation. *Addict. Behav.* **15,** 197–207.

[37]J. K. Bobo, L. D. Gilchrist, R. F. Schilling, B. Noach, and S. P. Schinke (1987) Cigarette smoking cessation attempts by recovering alcoholics. *Addict. Behav.* **12,** 209–215.

[38]J. K. Bobo, R. F. Schilling, L. D. Gilchrist, and S. P. Schinke (1986) The double triumph: sustained sobriety and successful cigarette smoking cessation. *J. Subst. Abuse Treat.* **3,** 2125.

[39]W. R. Miller, K. E. Hedrick, and C. A. Taylor (1983) Addictive behviors and life problems before and after behavioral treatment of problem drinkers. *Addict. Behav.* **8,** 403–412.

[40]B. M. Maletzky and J. Klotter (1974) Smoking and alcoholism. *Am. J. Psychiatry* **131,** 446,447.

[41]A. M. Joseph and K. L. Nichol (1990) The long-term effects of smoking intervention on drug dependency treatment program outcomes. *Clin. Res.* **38,** 696A.

[42]J. K. Bobo and L. D. Gilchrist (1983) Urging the alcoholic client to quit smoking cigarettes. *Addict. Behav.* **8,** 297–305.

[43]J. M. Knapp, C. L. Rosheim, and E. A. Meister Managing tobacco dependency in chemical dependency treatment facilities: A survey of current attitudes and policies (personal communication).

[44]V. C. Pletcher, L. S. Lysaght, and V. L. Hyman (1990) *Treating Nicotine Addiction: A Challenge for the Recovery Professional.* Hazelden Foundation, Center City, MN.

[45]D. E. Beauchamp (1990) Alcohol and tobacco as public health challenges in a democracy. *Br. J. Addict.* **85,** 251–254.

Buprenorphine for Opioid and Cocaine Dependence

Marc I. Rosen
and Thomas R. Kosten

Pharmacological treatment for opioid dependence currently employs one of two general approaches: maintenance with an opioid agonist such as methadone,[1] or detoxification and induction onto the opioid antagonist naltrexone. Buprenorphine is a mixed opioid agonist/antagonist that may help addicts for whom conventional detoxification or methadone-maintenance treatments are not effective.

There are several drawbacks to long-term methadone maintenance that may be ameliorated by buprenorphine maintenance. One is the difficulty terminating methadone maintenance because of the protracted withdrawal syndrome.[2,3] The second difficulty is the frequent abuse of cocaine by methadone-maintained patients. In this chapter we discuss three potential uses of buprenorphine:

1. Detoxification from opiates and induction onto naltrexone;
2. Treatment of opiate dependence; and
3. Treatment of cocaine-abusing opiate addicts.

From: *Drug and Alcohol Abuse Reviews, Vol. 4: Drug Abuse Treatment*
Ed: R. R. Watson

Pharmacological Considerations

Buprenorphine is a chemical hybrid of an opiate agonist, etorphine, and an opiate antagonist, diprenorphine. It is marketed as an analgesic—0.4 mg of im buprenorphine is equianalgesic with 10 mg of im morphine, with each providing approx 6 h of analgesia.[4] Buprenorphine binds to μ opiate receptors, but is thought to exert only partial agonist activity. Whether a dosage of buprenorphine acts physiologically as an agonist or antagonist depends on whether the patient is already opiate-dependent. A mixed opiate agonist–antagonist will precipitate withdrawal symptoms in opiate-dependent subjects, and it does not completely suppress abstinence symptoms in withdrawing high-dose, morphine-dependent subjects.[5] In opiate-naive subjects, buprenorphine acts as an agonist with opioid effects of analgesia, sedation, and miosis. Patients may complain of opioid agonist side effects: nausea, vomiting, sweating, and headache. However, sublingual doses of up to 32 mg produce no respiratory depression, making the risks of overdose low.[6]

Buprenorphine is thought to bind with a high affinity to opiate receptors and to disassociate slowly from the receptors. A placebo-controlled study showed that high doses of iv naloxone, up to 10 mg, were required to reverse buprenorphine-induced respiratory depression.[7] Unlike naloxone-precipitated withdrawal in morphine-treated patients, which is immediate, naloxone reversal of buprenorphine's effects took 3 h, suggesting a slow dissociation of buprenorphine from receptors. However, low doses of buprenorphine do not block the effects of concomitantly administered naloxone-precipitated withdrawal among opioid-dependent subjects, probably because of the slow onset of buprenorphine's action compared to naloxone.[8]

Sublingual buprenorphine is administered in an alcohol base that the patient holds under his or her tongue for 2 min. Sublingual buprenorphine has approximately two-thirds of the behavioral and physiological potency of the same dose administered sc.[9] Jasinski et al.[9] found the onset of miosis, euphoria, and drug liking was evident by 1 h after administration of both sublingual and sc buprenorphine. Peak changes in pupil diameter and behavioral effects occurred 3–4 h after buprenorphine administration. Single sublingual buprenorphine doses of up to 4 mg produced no significant changes in body temperature, blood pressure, or respiratory or heart rates, despite producing considerable subjective effects and changes in pupil diameter. Buprenorphine's high lipophilicity facilitates its entry into the central nervous system, and its plasma half-life is approx 3 h.[10] However, its behavioral effects are undoubtedly more dependent on central nervous system receptor binding than on plasma pharmacokinetics.

Buprenorphine for Opioid Detoxification

Detoxification from opiates can be accomplished in several ways: methadone stabilization and then taper,[2] clonidine detoxification,[11] and clonidine–naltrexone detoxification.[12] There are several drawbacks with any of these approaches. First, the patient must tolerate withdrawal symptoms for several days, leading to intense craving and potential illicit opiate use by outpatients during this time. Second, although clonidine has several advantages over methadone tapering, including no abuse liability, no need for special licensing, and little risk of overdose with appropriate monitoring, it has some limitations. Clonidine produces an unpleasant sedation and light headedness, and neither clonidine nor naltrexone is reinforcing.

Buprenorphine causes dependence in opiate-naive subjects. Early work with buprenorphine showed that 30 d of treatment of nonopiate-dependent subjects with 8 mg of sublingual buprenorphine produced a mild withdrawal syndrome when the buprenorphine was discontinued.[13] This relatively mild dependence induced by buprenorphine has been confirmed by other studies.[14]

One outpatient study[15] used a double-dummy, double-blind condition to compare outpatient detoxification of opioid addicts by stabilization for 3 wk on either 2 mg of sublingual buprenorphine or 30 mg of methadone daily, followed by 4 wk of gradual dosage reduction, followed by 6 wk of placebo medication. A repeated measures analysis of variance failed to reveal any significant differences between the buprenorphine- and methadone-maintained groups on any indices of drug use. Subject retention was equally poor with both treatments, especially after placebo substitution. The mean retention time for the buprenorphine group was 48½ d, which was not statistically significant from the mean duration for the methadone group.

One method for opioid detoxification using buprenorphine would be to stabilize opioid-dependent patients on buprenorphine and then switch them to naltrexone. We have shown that heroin addicts can be stabilized on buprenorphine at doses of 2–6 mg sublingually daily with minimal withdrawal symptoms.[16,17] In our month-long study of heroin- and methadone-dependent addicts, 28 of the 39 subjects remained on buprenorphine. Withdrawal symtpoms for all dosages of buprenorphine were mild, the lowest initial withdrawal symptoms being at the lowest (2 mg) buprenorphine dose. The higher 3–6 mg buprenorphine doses initially triggered more withdrawal symptoms that decreased over the next 2 wk. Twenty-three of the patients on buprenorphine after 1 mo were discontinued from buprenorphine and, on successive days, given naltrexone in doses of 1, 6, 12.5, and 50 mg with minimal withdrawal symptoms.

Thus, an alternative to the gradual buprenorphine taper in Bickel's study would be stabilization on buprenorphine, followed by abrupt detoxification onto naltrexone. Our clinical experience is that detoxification from buprenorphine and induction onto naltrexone are easier than detoxification from methadone and induction onto naltrexone. We compared the withdrawal symptoms of five addicts who had been maintained on 3 mg of buprenorphine sublingually for 1 mo in the aforementioned study to patients abruptly withdrawn from methadone.[18] These five were then discontinued from buprenorphine by blinded placebo substitution and underwent a placebo-controlled, double-blind challenge with iv naloxone at 0.5 mg/kg. The mean peak severity of withdrawal was 15 (SD = 4.1) out of a possible full Abstinence Rating Scale score of 45. By comparison, the mean severity of withdrawal precipitated by 1 mg of naltrexone in a group of 15 methadone-maintained patients (mean dose = 35 mg)[19] was 22 (SD = 9.3). Five hours after the buprenorphine-maintained patients underwent the naloxone challenge, oral naltrexone was given at either 12.5 or 25 mg without precipitating further withdrawal symptoms. On the following day, the naltrexone dose was doubled, resulting in some sleep difficulty, but no major withdrawal symptoms.

Maintenance Buprenorphine Treatment for Opioid Addiction

Like methadone, maintenance buprenorphine treatment should act to reduce craving, maintain patients in treatment by its reinforcing properties, and block the effects of illicit opioids. This latter property has been studied in several experimental paradigms. Jasinski et al.[13] showed that a daily dose of 8 mg of buprenorphine blocked the effects of 120 mg of im morphine for 1½ h after buprenorphine and blocked 30 mg of morphine given 29 h after the last dose of buprenorphine. In the previously described study of Bickel et al.,[15] the buprenorphine- and methadone-maintained patients were each administered a 6 mg im injection of hydromorphone. Thirty milligrams of methadone attenuated the effects of this challenge dose to a greater extent than did buprenorphine on both physiologic (pupil constriction) and self report measures. Bickel et al.[20] used a within-subjects design to show that there is a buprenorphine dose-related blockade of im hydromorphone by buprenorphine maintenance. The same patients maintained on 2 mg of buprenorphine for 2 wk had a mean "high" of 4 (on an analog scale from 1–10) after a cumulative dose of 18 mg of hydromorphone, but this "high" was halved by maintenance of these same patients on 8 mg of buprenorphine for 2 wk. We have preliminary data showing that this blockade of opioid effects in patients maintained on 12-mg doses of buprenorphine lasts at least 3 d after discontinuation of buprenorphine.[21]

Equally relevant to buprenorphine's therapeutic potential is its ability to decrease opiate craving, the desire of an addict to seek out heroin actively. Mello et al.[22] examined this property of buprenorphine in hospitalized, detoxified opiate addicts who were maintained on either buprenorphine, 8 mg sc daily, or placebo. Addicts were able to work at a button-pushing task for either money or heroin. Buprenorphine-maintained addicts chose to self-administer only 2–31% of the available heroin, whereas placebo-maintained addicts took 93–100% of the available heroin. These results were corroborated by the finding in monkeys that buprenorphine, at doses that do not suppress food intake, suppressed hydromorphone self-administration.[23] The direct clinical relevance of this finding is unclear, since it occurred at a buprenorphine dose equivalent to 24–48 mg daily in humans, and methadone, which is known to be clinically efficacious, did not suppress opiate self-administration at the tested dosages.

Buprenorphine for Cocaine Abuse

Pure μ agonists, such as methadone and morphine, do not attenuate cocaine euphoria. Coadministration of iv morphine (0–10 mg) and cocaine (0–32 mg) to nonopiate-dependent subjects yields "highs" that are equal to or greater than, but never less than, the "high" from either cocaine or morphine administered separately.[24] These data are supported by the clinical observation that patients commonly inject "speedballs," comprised of a combination of cocaine and heroin. Data from our methadone program suggest that methadone treatment does not reduce cocaine use for many opiate addicts, perhaps because methadone makes cocaine use more pleasurable. A 2½-yr followup of 142 patients consecutively admitted to methadone maintenance in 1980 showed that 66 patients used more cocaine after 2.5 yr on methadone, only 36 patients used less, and just 40 did not use cocaine.[25] A critical minority of patients on methadone maintenance progressed from relatively infrequent cocaine abuse to daily cocaine abuse on methadone.

In a recent review, Johanson and Fischman state: "Place preference and self-stimulation techniques suggest that the reinforcing effects of stimulants and opiates have overlapping mechanisms and sites of action."[26] Preclinical evidence suggests that buprenorphine may not interact with cocaine the way pure μ agonists do. Rats maintained on 1 wk of buprenorphine show an attenuated cocaine-conditioned place preference when compared with saline-treated rats.[27] The buprenorphine-treated rats showed a >50% reduction in their preference for the side of the cage associated with cocaine administration. Another paradigm examined the effect of buprenorphine treatment on rhesus monkeys taught to self-administer iv cocaine.[28] Five rhesus monkeys maintained on chronic buprenorphine treatment at 0.7 mg/kg/d suppressed their cocaine self-administration to between 91–97% of their baseline levels of self-administration. This reduction in cocaine self-administration was dose-dependent with lesser reductions at smaller dosages of buprenorphine. There was some suppression of food intake at these doses of buprenorphine, which was not believed to be behaviorally or nutritionally significant. Since conditioned place preference depends on classical conditioning mechanisms and self-administration is an operant conditioning paradigm, these two convergent studies support buprenorphine's potential efficacy in reducing cocaine's reinforcing properties.

We have compared the effects of intranasal cocaine given alone and given in combination with buprenorphine in five opiate- and cocaine-addicted patients.[29] Buprenorphine maintenance at a dosage of 2 mg daily did not attenuate cocaine effects compared to placebo treatment. Instead, buprenorphine increased baseline and cocaine-induced elevations in "high," "pleasant," pulse, and blood pressure. Enhancement of cocaine effects by short-term dosing with 2 mg of sublingual buprenorphine suggests a "speedball"-like interaction between low-dose buprenorphine and cocaine.

A similar study by Teoh et al.[30] compared the response to 30 mg of iv cocaine in 16 opiate-dependent patients after detoxification from opioids and after 2 wk of maintenance on buprenorphine. Preliminary data suggest that the eight patients maintained on 4 mg buprenorphine rated the quality of cocaine's pleasant effects slightly lower after 2 wk of buprenorphine treatment, whereas the eight patients maintained on 8 mg of buprenorphine rated the cocaine effect slightly more enhanced after 2 wk of buprenorphine treatment. Thus, challenge studies confirm that buprenorphine does not "block" the cocaine high, but the studies do not address the question of whether cocaine interacts differently with buprenorphine than methadone.

A 1-mo open clinical trial of buprenorphine in 41 opioid addicts was extremely promising.[31] These patients were compared to 61 patients on methadone maintenance. The rate of heroin-positive urine tests from weekly toxicology screening was 33% for addicts on methadone and 37% for addicts on buprenorphine, roughly equivalent. However, the rate of cocaine-positive urine toxicologies in the methadone-maintained patients was 24% compared with only 3% among addicts on buprenorphine. Six cocaine-using "crossover" patients who had been maintained on methadone were switched over to buprenorphine in this study. Five of these six patients stopped using cocaine completely during the month that they were on buprenorphine, and the sixth substantially reduced his cocaine use. Higher buprenorphine doses (as high as 8 mg) were associated with fewer cocaine-positive urine tests.

Controlled studies have been less promising. Johnson and Fudala randomized 162 opiate-dependent patients to 3 mo of treatment with either buprenorphine 8 mg, methadone 20 mg, or methadone 60 mg daily, administered in a double-blind, double-dummy technique.[32,33] Treatment retention for the 119-d maintenance period was only 40% for the buprenorphine group and 37% for the 60-mg methadone group, and was even worse, only 20%, for the methadone 20-mg group. There was a trend toward fewer opiate-positive urines on buprenorphine, 37%, compared with 49% on methadone 60 mg and 64% on methadone 20 mg. The overall rate of cocaine-positive urines was 57% over the 17-wk study without any significant difference between groups in any week. The poor retention in this study and minimal psychotherapy may have attenuated a subtle effect favoring buprenorphine in combination with psychotherapy.

We have used a similar paradigm to compare buprenorphine at 2 mg and 6 mg sublingually to methadone at 35 mg and 65 mg during a 24-wk trial in 125 opioid-dependent patients.[34] The average retention was 18 ± 7 wk with lower retention in the buprenorphine than in the methadone groups (15.5 vs 20 wk). Urine toxicology for opioids averaged 68% in the buprenorphine group and 43% in the methadone group, which was significantly different. Maximum reduction of cocaine abuse in any one week (this occurred during weeks 10–13 for all groups) was greater for the 6-mg buprenorphine group than the 2-mg buprenorphine group (71 vs 28%), and the methadone groups had an intermediate reduction at 40%. The overall rate of cocaine abuse was 47% with no significant differences across treatment groups at baseline. Thus, higher doses of buprenorphine appear to be more efficacious than lower doses of buprenorphine for reducing cocaine abuse.

Conclusion

Buprenorphine is a mixed opiate agonist–antagonist that slowly dissociates from opiate receptors. These properties suggest a potential role for buprenorphine in opiate detoxification, and we have found this to be a useful treatment. Buprenorphine effectively minimizes opiate craving in addicts and blocks the effect of exogenously administered opiates. The interaction of buprenorphine and cocaine is more complex, and appears to depend on several factors, including duration of buprenorphine treatment, dosage of buprenorphine, and what the cocaine–buprenorphine combination is being compared to.

The preliminary data suggest that higher buprenorphine dosages are a more effective treatment for cocaine and opiate use, but more testing needs to be done in this area, especially in the 8–12 mg daily dosage range. There have not been any crossover studies between buprenorphine and methadone to determine if individual characteristics predict an addict's response to one drug or another. Clinical trials will also need to focus on potential augmentation strategies, e.g., desipramine augmentation for cocaine-addicted opiate addicts. Ultimately, there may be a complex answer to the question of whether buprenorphine is a better treatment for drug addiction than methadone.

Acknowledgments

This research was supported by grants from the National Institute on Drug Abuse to T. R. Kosten: P50-DA04060, R18-DA06190, ROI-DA05626, and K02-DA00112.

References

[1]J. R. Cooper, F. Altman, B. S. Brown, and D. Czechowicz (1983) *Research on the Treatment of Narcotic Addiction.* National Institute of Mental Health, Rockville, MD.

[2]P. Cushman and V. P. Dole (1973) Detoxification of methadone maintenance patients. *JAMA* **226,** 747–751.

[3]E. C. Senay, W. Dorus, F. Goldberg, and W. Thornton (1977) Withdrawal from methadone maintenance. *Arch. Gen. Psychiatry* **34,** 361–367.

[4]G. A. Gilman, L. S. Goodman, T. W. Rall, and F. Murad (eds.) (1985) *The Pharmacological Basis of Therapeutics.* 7th ed. Macmillan, New York.

[5]R. W. Houde (1979) Analgesic effectiveness of the narcotic agonist–antagonists. *Br. J. Clin. Pharmacol.* **7,** 297S–308S.

[6]S. L. Walsh, K. L. Preston, M. L. Stitzer, G. E. Bigelow, and I. A. Liebson (1991) The acute effects of high dose buprenorphine in non-dependent humans. *Proceedings of the Committee on Problems of Drug Dependence 1991.* L.S. Harris, ed. National Institute on Drug Abuse, Rockville, MD, in press.

[7]T. J. Gal (1989) Naloxone reversal of buprenorphine–induced respiratory depression. *Clin. Pharmacol. Ther.* **45,** 66–71.

[8]K. L. Preston, G. E. Bigelow, and I. A. Liebson (1988) Buprenorphine and naloxone alone and in combination in opioid-dependent humans. *Psychopharmacology* **44,** 484–490.

[9]D. R. Jasinski, P. J. Fudala, and R. E. Johnson (1989) Sublingual versus subcutaneous buprenorphine in opiate abusers. *Clin. Pharm. Ther.* **45,** 513–519.

[10]J. W. Louis (1985) Buprenorphine. *Drug Alcohol Depend.* **14,** 363–372.

[11]M. S. Gold, D. E. Redmond, and H. D. Kleber (1978) Clonidine in opiate withdrawal. *Lancet* **1,** 929,930.

[12]E. Vining, T. R. Kosten, and H. D. Kleber (1988) Clinical utility of rapid clonidine-naltrexone detoxification for opioid abusers. *Br. J. Addict.* **83,** 567–575.

[13]D. R. Jasinski, J. S. Pevnick, and J. D. Griffith (1978) Human pharmacology and abuse potential of the analgesic buprenorphine. *Arch. Gen. Psychiatry* **35,** 501–516.

[14]J. E. Dum, J. Blasig, and A. Herz (1981) Buprenorphine: physical dependence and liability. *Eur. J. Pharmacol.* **70,** 293–300.

[15]W. K. Bickel, M. L. Stitzer, G. E. Bigelow, I. A. Liebson, P. R. Jasinski, and

R. E. Johnson (1988) A clinical trial of buprenorphine: Comparison with methadone in the detoxification of heroin addicts. *Clin. Pharmacol. Ther.* **43,** 72–78.

[16]T. R. Kosten and H. D. Kleber (1988) Buprenorphine detoxification from opioid dependence. *Life Sci.* **42,** 635–641.

[17]T. R. Kosten, C. Morgan, and H. D. Kleber (1991) Treatment of heroin addicts using buprenorphine. *Am. J. Drug Alcohol Abuse* **17(2),** 119–228.

[18]T. R. Kosten New approaches for rapid detoxification and induction onto naltrexone. *Adv. Alcohol. Subst. Abuse,* in press.

[19]D. S. Charney, D. E. Redmond, M. P. Galloway, H. D. Kleber, G. R. Heninger, M. Murberg, and R. H. Roth (1984) Naltrexone precipitated opiate withdrawal in methadone addicted human subjects: evidence for moradrenergic hypoactivity. *Life Sci.* **35,** 1263–1272.

[20]W. K. Bickel, M. L. Stitzer, G. E. Bigelow, I. A. Liebson, D. R. Jasinksi, and R. E. Johnson (1988) Buprenorphine dose related blockade of opioid challenge effects in opioid dependent humans. *J. Pharm. Exp. Ther.* **247,** 47–53.

[21]E. A. Wallace, M. I. Rosen, H. R. Pearsall, S. W. Woods, L. H. Price, C. J. McDougle, and T. R. Kosten (1992) Buprenorphine: duration of blockade of effects of intramuscular opioids. Committee on the Problems of Drug Dependence 1992, submitted abstract.

[22]N. K. Mello, J. H. Mendelson, and U. C. Kuehnle (1982) Buprenorphine effects on human heroin self-administration: an operant analysis. *J. Pharmacol. Exp. Ther.* **223(1),** 30–39.

[23]J. H. Mendelson (1983) Comparison of buprenorphine and methadone effects on opiate self-administration in primates. *J. Pharmacol. Exp. Ther.* **225(2),** 378–386.

[24]R. W. Foltin and M. W. Fischmann (1990) *The Cardiovascular and Subjective Affects of Intravenous Cocaine and Morphine Combinations ("Speedballs") in Humans.* American College of Neuropsychopharmacology.

[25]T. R. Kosten, B. J. Rounsaville, and H. D. Kleber (1988) Antecedents and consequences of cocaine abuse among opioid addicts: a 2.5 year follow up. *J. Nerv. Men. Disease* **176,** 176–181.

[26]C. E. Johanson and M. W. Fischman (1989) The pharmacology of cocaine related to its abuse. *Pharmacol. Rev.* **41(1),** 3–52.

[27]T. A. Kosten, D. W. Marby, and E. J. Nestler (1991) Chronic buprenorphine attenuates cocaine conditioned placed preference, in *Proceedings of the Committee on Problems of Drug Dependence 1991.* L. S. Harris, ed. National Institute on Drug Abuse, Rockville, MD, in press.

[28]N. K. Mello, J. H. Mendelson, M. B. Bree, and S. E. Lukas (1989) Buprenorphine suppresses cocaine self-administration by Rhesus monkeys. *Science* **245,** 859–862.

[29]M. I. Rosen, H. R. Pearsall, C. J. McDougle, L. H. Price, S. W. Woods, and

T. R. Kosten (1992) Effects of acute buprenorphine on responses to intranasal cocaine. *Proceedings of the Committee on the Problems of Drug Dependence 1992,* submitted abstract.

[30]S. K. Teoh, P. Sintavanarong, J. Kuehnle, J. H. Mendelson, E. Hallring, E. Rhoades, and N. K. Mello (1991) Buprenorphine effects on morphine and cocaine challenges in heroin and cocaine dependent men, in *Proceedings of the Committee on Problems of Drug Dependence 1991.* L. S. Harris, ed. National Institute on Drug Abuse, Rockville, MD, in press.

[31]T. R. Kosten, H. D. Kleber, and C. Morgan (1989) Treatment of cocaine abuse with buprenorphine. *Biol. Psychiatry* **26,** 637–639.

[32]R. E. Johnson, P. J. Fudala, and J. H. Jaffey (1990) Outpatient comparison of buprenorphine and methadone maintenance. I. Effects on opiate use and self–reported adverse effects and withdrawal symptomatology, in *Proceedings of the Committee on Problems of Drug Dependence 1991.* L. S. Harris, ed. National Institute on Drug Abuse, Rockville, MD, pp. 585,586.

[33]P. J. Fudala, R. E. Johnson, and J. H. Jaffey (1990) Outpatient comparison of buprenorphine and methadone maintenance. II. Effects on cocaine usage, retention time and study and missed clinic visits, in *Proceedings of the Committee on Problems of Drug Dependence 1991.* L. S. Harris, ed. National Institute on Drug Abuse, Rockville, MD, pp. 587,588.

[34]T. R. Kosten, R. S. Schottenfeld, C. H. Morgan, J. Falcioni, and D. Ziedonis (1991) Buprenorphine vs methadone for opioid and cocaine dependence, in *Proceedings of the Committee on Problems of Drug Dependence 1991.* L. S. Harris, ed. National Institute on Drug Abuse, Rockville, MD, in press.

Carbamazepine in the Treatment of Cocaine-Induced Disorders

Clinical and Mechanistic Implications

Susan R. B. Weiss, Robert M. Post, and Thomas G. Aigner

Carbamazepine is one of the most potent anticonvulsants against completed amygdala-kindled seizures, with no impact, however, on the development of these seizures in the rat. Based on this observation and the finding that lidocaine-kindled seizures produce marked increases in behavioral aggression in the rat,[1–3] we wished to examine whether carbamazepine would be able to block these aggressive responses, presumably in the absence of its ability to block the local anesthetic seizure. Contrary to our expectations, carbamazepine was highly effective in blocking the development of both lidocaine- and cocaine-kindled seizures.[4–7]

Given these observations, and the well-known anticonvulsant and positive psychotropic effects of carbamazepine in the treatment of patients with seizure disorders and manic-depressive illness, we began to consider the potential utility of carbamazepine in the treatment of cocaine abuse, and its associated behavioral and convulsive side effects. As illustrated in Table 1, carbamazepine is effective in some aspects of cocaine's behavioral pharma-

From: *Drug and Alcohol Abuse Reviews, Vol. 4: Drug Abuse Treatment*
Ed: R. R. Watson

Table 1
Differential Pharmacotherapy of Development vs Expression of Cocaine-Induced Behavioral Sensitization

	Development	Expression
DA antagonists		
haloperidol		
(0.2 mg/kg)	++	0
(0.5 mg/kg)	++	0
DA_1 SCH 23390	++	0
DA_2 raclopride	++	0
α_2 agonist		
clonidine	++	++
Benzodiazepine α_2 agonist		
diazepam	++	++
Lithium	++	?
Carbamazepine	0	0

cological profile, but not others. These might be important clues not only to the mechanism of action of carbamazepine, but also to the differential mechanisms underlying different aspects of cocaine abuse syndromes. Carbamazepine is ineffective in blocking the acute effects of psychomotor stimulants in animals and humans.[8,9] Since the acute psychomotor stimulant properties of cocaine and its sensitization mechanisms have been most closely linked to dopaminergic systems, and cocaine self-administration has also been linked to this neurotransmitter system, it was unclear whether carbamazepine would be able to inhibit cocaine self-administration. Carbamazepine was found to decrease cocaine self-administration in rhesus monkeys,[10] further raising the question of whether it might also be associated with positive therapeutic effects in the clinic. In this chapter, we review the effects of carbamazepine on each aspect of the evolving cocaine syndromes and discuss the potential mechanisms that may underlie its differential impact on these target areas.

Effects of Carbamazepine on Cocaine-Kindled Seizures and Associated Lethality

As illustrated in Fig. 1, when carbamazepine is administered in the diet (5 g carbamazepine/kg food) in order to achieve clinically relevant blood levels,[11] it is highly effective in blocking the development of cocaine-kindled

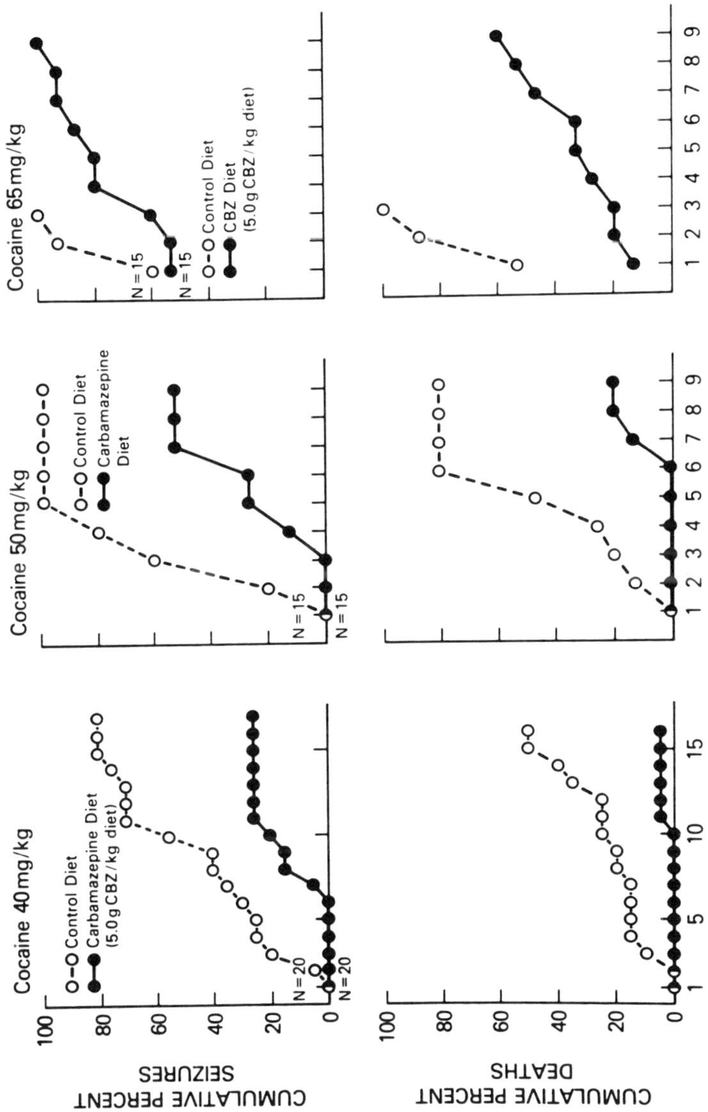

Fig. 1. Chronic carbamazepine prevents the development of cocaine-kindled seizures and mortality.

seizures (Fig. 1, top). When animals were given cocaine (40 mg/kg, ip) on a once-daily basis, 80% of the animals showed seizures in the first 2 wk of treatment, and this was reduced to less than 25% in animals treated with the carbamazepine diet. At a higher dose of cocaine, 50 mg/kg, kindled seizure evolution occurs more rapidly, and the carbamazepine diet is still able to reduce cocaine seizures (Fig. 1, top) and their associated lethality Fig. 1, bottom). For example, while 80% of the animals administered cocaine with the control diet had died by d 6, none of the animals treated with the carbamazepine diet had died at this time, even though several had experienced cocaine seizures. At the highest dose of cocaine tested (65 mg/kg, ip), all of the control-diet-treated animals had seizures and died in the first 3 d, whereas 50% survived with carbamazepine treatment. Thus, these data illustrate the high degree of effectiveness of chronic oral administration of carbamazepine in blocking the development of cocaine-kindled seizures and in preventing their associated lethality.

Despite the marked effects of chronic oral carbamazepine in the diet on cocaine and lidocaine kindling, intermittent ip administration of carbamazepine is either without effect or worsens the cocaine-induced seizures and lethality.[6] A series of studies have demonstrated that this is not owing to inadequate dosage, blood levels, or pretreatment time prior to cocaine administration. When administered once daily prior to cocaine, low (5 mg/kg, ip) or moderate (15 mg/kg, ip) doses of carbamazepine were ineffective, whereas higher doses (50 mg/kg, ip) actually exacerbated cocaine kindling. Carbamazepine treatment (50 mg/kg, ip) 5 h before cocaine, in order to achieve blood levels similar to those achieved with the carbamazepine diet (in which the -10,11-epoxide metabolite predominates), was also without effect on cocaine kindling. Treatment regimens of 3 wk with 15 or 50 mg/kg, ip, of carbamazepine before and during the initiation of cocaine kindling also were ineffective and, at the higher dose, enhanced cocaine kindling, indicating it was not the duration of intermittent treatment that accounted for its lack of efficacy.

As a final assessment of whether this lack of efficacy could be related to route of administration rather than intermittency, we had animals eating all of their carbamazepine diet within a restricted period of time: 2 h/d. This manipulation was also effective against cocaine kindling. However, when we determined blood levels of carbamazepine and its epoxide metabolite 24 h after the last dose, detectable levels of each were still observed. Thus, even this intermittent feeding regime provided some degree of continuous drug availability that was sufficient to attenuate cocaine kindling.

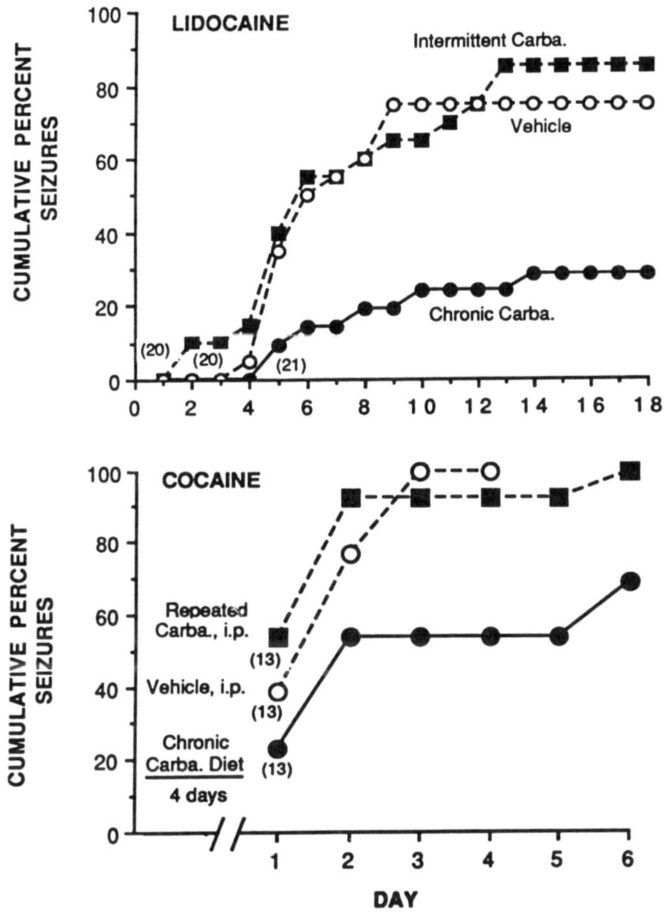

Fig. 2. Chronic carbamazepine is required to block local-anesthetic-kindled seizures.

A similar dysjunction is observed in the ability of carbamazepine to inhibit local anesthetic-kindled seizures with lidocaine. That is, chronic oral carbamazepine is highly effective in blocking lidocaine-kindled seizures, but repeated intermittent carbamazepine (15 mg/kg) is without effect (Fig. 2). Taken together, these data suggest that there are different biological processes that are induced with chronic compared with repeated intermittent administration of carbamazepine that are important to its effect. Elsewhere,[12–16] we have discussed that this local-anesthetic seizure model system may be an interesting paradigm for dissecting possible effects of carbamazepine

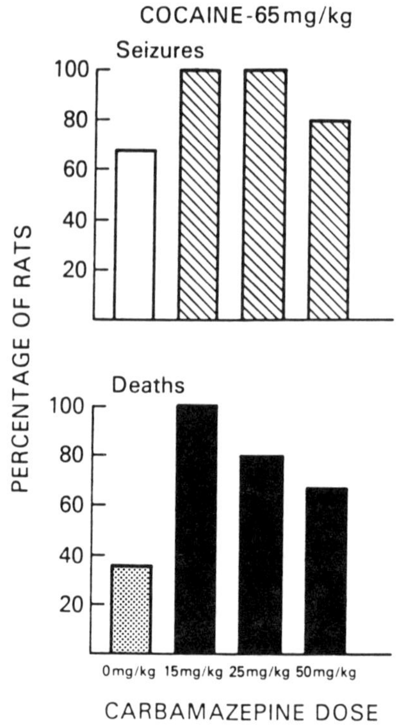

Fig. 3. Lack of effect of acute carbamazepine on cocaine-induced seizures and lethality.

that may be related to its long-term psychotropic effects in manic-depressive illness. In the treatment of mania and depression, chronic drug administration also appears to be important to its therapeutic efficacy, which occurs with a lag of some 2–4 wk before maximum clinical effectiveness is observed.

Although chronic carbamazepine is highly effective in the blockade of local anesthetic-kindled seizure evolution, once these seizures have become fully kindled or if an acute high-dose seizure is produced, as illustrated in Fig. 3, carbamazepine (administered either acutely or chronically) is not effective. These data suggest that carbamazepine is acting on processes underlying local anesthetic kindling evolution or development rather than on processes related to the full-blown seizure *per se*. It is noteworthy that these data provide a double dissociation with amygdala-kindled seizures, where carbamazepine shows the opposite pattern; it is ineffective in the development phase, but highly effective in completed seizures.[17]

Carbamazepine's Effects on Acute Psychomotor Stimulant Administration and Behavioral Sensitization

As illustrated in Fig. 4, carbamazepine is ineffective in blocking acute locomotor hyperactivity achieved by cocaine. These data parallel similar data with amphetamine,[18] and are consistent with the clinical data of Meyendorff et al.[8] that carbamazepine is unable to block the euphoria associated with methylphenidate administration in humans or the high associated with smoked cocaine.[9] The mood-elevating effects in humans and locomotor-activating effects in animals are thought to be similarly mediated. In marked contrast, dopamine receptor-blocking agents, such as the neuroleptics, are highly effective in blocking cocaine and amphetamine-induced locomotor activation.[19]

Carbamazepine is ineffective in blocking cocaine-induced behavioral sensitization achieved either by repeated cocaine (10 mg/kg, ip once daily, Fig. 4) or by a single high dose of cocaine (40 mg/kg ip) followed by a low dose challenge[7] (Figs. 5A and 5B). These data are particularly interesting, since both cocaine's acute effects and its effects on sensitization have been linked to dopaminergic mechanisms, particularly those involving the nucleus accumbens.[21,22] We have demonstrated that depletions of dopamine in the nucleus accumbens, even those insufficient to block the acute locomotor-activating effects of cocaine, are able to inhibit context-dependent behavioral sensitization.[23,24] Similarly, electrolytic and dopaminergic lesions of the amygdala are able to block context-dependent behavioral sensitization.[25] Thus, the inability of carbamazepine to block either the acute or sensitization effects of cocaine indicates that it does not have classical dopamine antagonist properties either similar to neuroleptics or to the effect of dopaminergic lesions in the mesolimbic areas of brain.

However, when high doses of cocaine (40 mg/kg, ip) are administered repeatedly in order to observe the evolution of stereotypy (and seizures), a partial effect of carbamazepine is observed.[7] The drug is insufficient to block the sensitization to stereotypy *per se,* although the peak degrees of stereotypy are consistently reduced during carbamazepine administration compared with vehicle control injections, as illustrated in Fig. 6A. This suggests that some component of carbamazepine's action is able to interact with striatal dopaminergic mechanisms that are thought to be important in stimulant-induced stereotypy, although carbamazepine was not able to inhibit the sen-

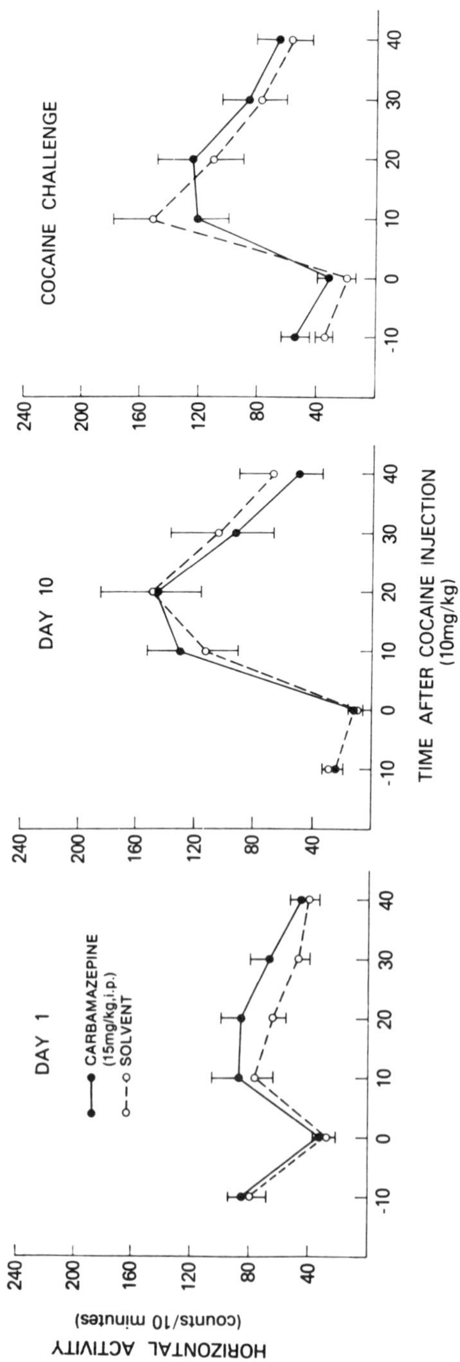

Fig. 4. Lack of effect of carbamazepine on cocaine-induced behavioral sensitization.

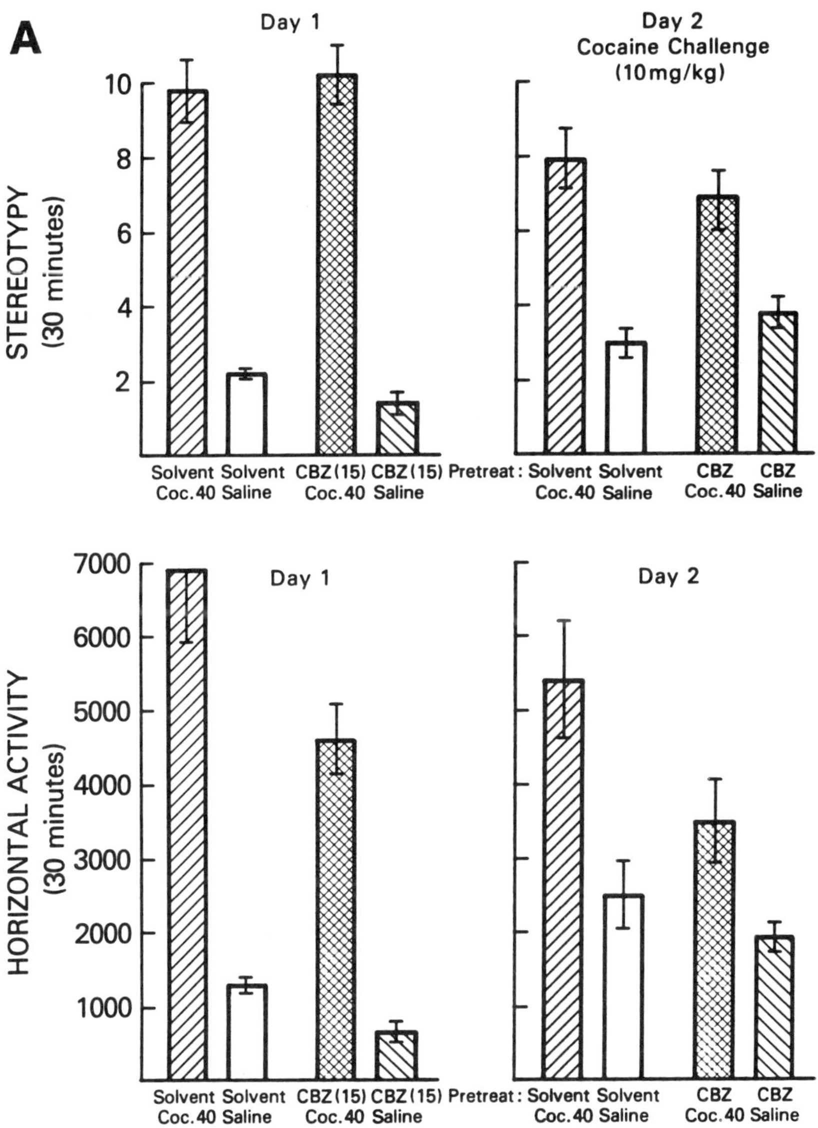

Fig. 5A. Lack of effect of acute carbamazepine on the development of cocaine sensitization.

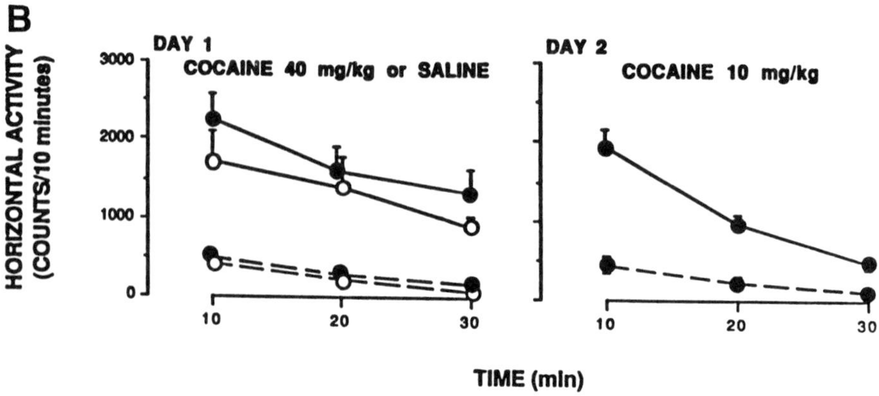

Fig. 5B. Chronic carbamazepine does not inhibit cocaine-induced hyperactivity (d 1) or sensitization (d 2). Day 1 treatment: COC 40 mg/kg (○—○ [control diet], ●—● [carbamazepine diet, 5.0 g/kg diet]) and saline (○- -○ [control diet], ●- -● [carbamazepine diet, 5.0 g/kg diet]).

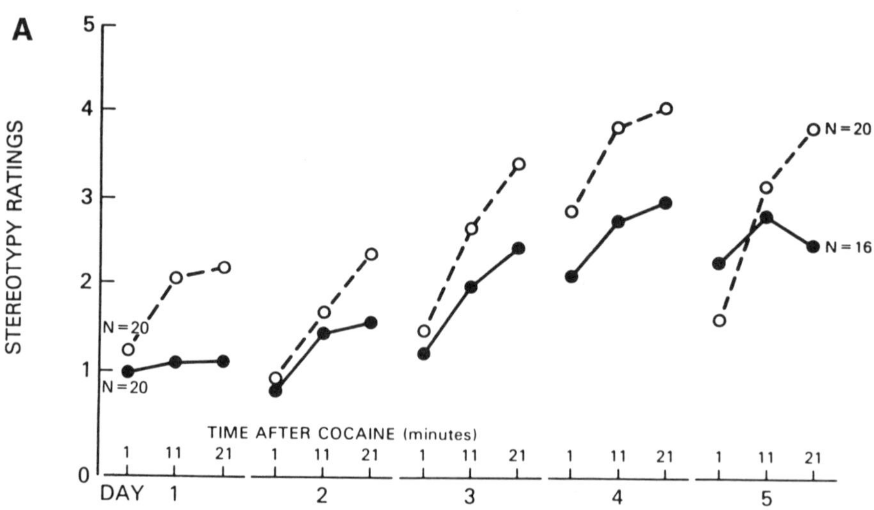

Fig. 6A. Carbamazepine decreases peak cocaine-induced stereotypy. ○- -○ Control diet; ●—● carbamazepine diet.

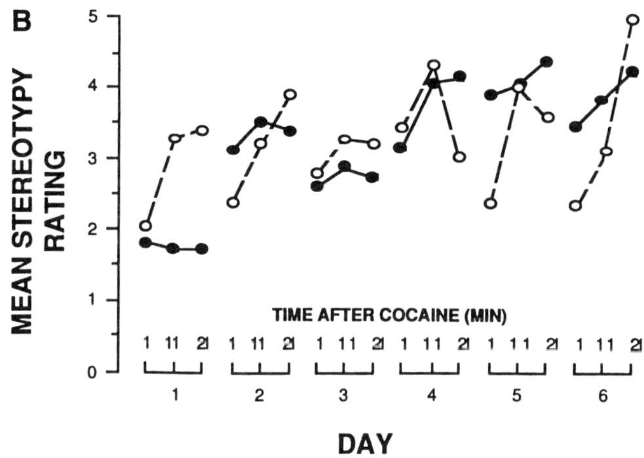

Fig. 6B. Lack of effect of carbamazepine on cocaine (50 mg/kg)-induced stereotypy. O- -O Control diet; ●—● carbamazepine diet (5.0 g/kg diet).

sitization effect. Moreover, at higher doses of cocaine (50 mg/kg; Fig. 6B), carbamazepine becomes ineffective even in blocking peak stereotypy as well as sensitization.[7]

Effects of Carbamazepine on Cocaine Self-Administration

Given the lack of effect of carbamazepine on the acute and sensitizing effects of cocaine, and the close linkage of psychomotor stimulant self-administration to dopaminergic mechanisms in the nucleus accumbens, one might have predicted that carbamazepine would be ineffective in the blockade of cocaine self-administration. Selective lesions of dopamine in the nucleus accumbens have previously been demonstrated to inhibit the iv self-administration of both amphetamine and cocaine.[22,26–29] We had postulated that carbamazepine could be a useful drug in the treatment of cocaine-induced disorders, based on its ability to inhibit cocaine-kindled seizures and their associated lethality[6] as reviewed earlier. We surmised that, even if the drug did not block the psychomotor stimulant properties of cocaine, it might nonetheless be useful in blocking some of cocaine's side effects, such as seizure evolution, or some of its psychiatric sequele, such as panic attacks, as discussed later. Since carbamazepine was effective in inhibiting

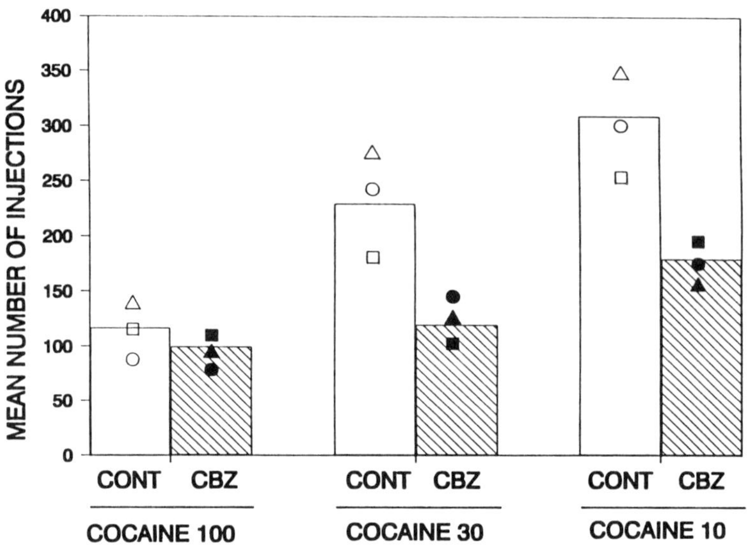

Fig. 7. Carbamazepine attenuates cocaine self-administration in rhesus monkeys. ■ = M1; ● = M2; ▲ = M3.

the paroxysmal components of cocaine-kindled seizures and their evolution, and paroxysmal pain syndromes, we postulated that it might also be effective in altering cocaine's stimulus or rewarding properties, even if it did not block cocaine's psychomotor stimulant effects. Thus, we undertook studies in rhesus monkeys to determine the effects of carbamazepine on cocaine self-administration.

Aigner and associates[10] found that orally administered carbamazepine in the diet attenuated cocaine self-administration in rhesus monkeys. When the carbamazepine diet was replaced by conventional diet, high rates of self-administration again resumed, as illustrated in Fig. 7. This is a representative animal of the three so far studied, demonstrating the consistent effect of carbamazepine on cocaine self-administration. In this study, rhesus monkeys were fitted with chronic indwelling iv catheters and allowed 2 h daily access to cocaine. Each animal was placed in a restraint chair in front of a computer monitor that had a touch-sensitive screen, so that the animal could obtain a 1-mL infusion of cocaine by touching any location on the screen 10 times. The carbamazepine diet contained 5 g carbamazepine/kg food, and the animals were given access to food 2 h each day prior to access to cocaine. Carbamazepine's effects on cocaine self-administration were evaluated at three doses of infusion: 100 µg/kg/mL, 30 µg/kg/mL, and 10 µg/kg/mL. Levels of carbamazepine and its -10,11-epoxide achieved by the diet in rhesus monkeys were similar to those in the low therapeutic range achieved in humans. Mean carbamazepine levels in the three rhesus monkeys were 4.41 µg/mL, and the epoxide was 0.5 µg/mL, yielding a combined total dose of carbamazepine and epoxide of 5.26 µg/mL (unpublished data of M. Clark). In clinical studies, the therapeutic range of carbamazepine is usually between 4 and 12 µg/mL, with an additional approx 25% contributed by -10,11-epoxide.

Oral administration of carbamazepine consistently diminished cocaine self-administration at the 30 and 10 µg/kg/mL infusion doses, but less consistently affected doses of 100 µg/kg/mL. At the 30 and 10 µg/kg/mL doses, basal rates of cocaine self-administration were substantially higher than those observed at the 100 µg/kg/mL dose. Thus, carbamazepine may have had rate-dependent effects, lowering cocaine self-administration associated with high rates, but being less effective at the lower rates of self-administration. The overall effect of carbamazepine in the three monkeys, studied at different doses per infusion and achieving different rates of cocaine self-administration, is illustrated in Figs. 8A, B, and C. The substantial ability of carbamazepine to reduce cocaine intake in these animals was observed without signs of behavioral sedation. The animals generally displayed similar degrees of stimulant-induced behavior as on the control diet despite decreased cocaine intake. Carroll et al.[30] found that carbamazepine decreased cocaine self-administration in rats, particularly those with high rates of self-administration. Since they did not manipulate the infusion dose, the higher rates of responding were also associated with greater cocaine intake in that study. However, Carroll et al.[30] also found a potentiation of cocaine's toxic effects (seizures and death) by carbamazepine and a decrease in cocaine-induced motor activity. This is also in contrast to our data in rats presented above, where carbamazepine did not inhibit activity and did reduce toxicity; i.e., both seizures and lethality. Carbamazepine was also well tolerated in our studies of rhesus monkey cocaine self-administration. One possible reason for this discrepancy is that the rats in the Carroll et al.[30] study self-administered cocaine over a 24-h period, which, in some cases, resulted in extremely high total cocaine doses of 200 mg/kg/d. Thus, it is possible that the animals succumbed to cocaine at a time when

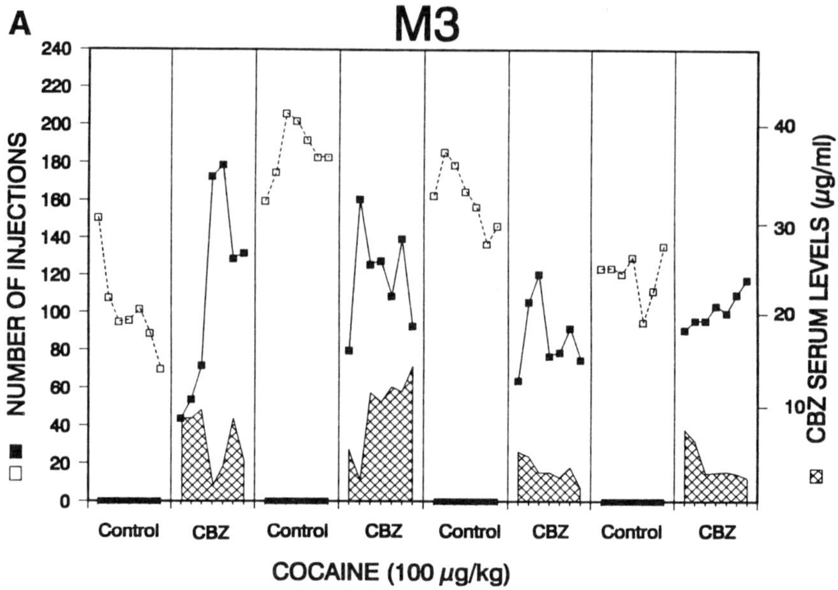
A
M3
240
220
200
180
160
140
120
100
80
60
40
20
0
NUMBER OF INJECTIONS
40
30
20
10
CBZ SERUM LEVELS (μg/ml)
Control
CBZ
Control
CBZ
Control
CBZ
Control
CBZ
COCAINE (100 μg/kg)

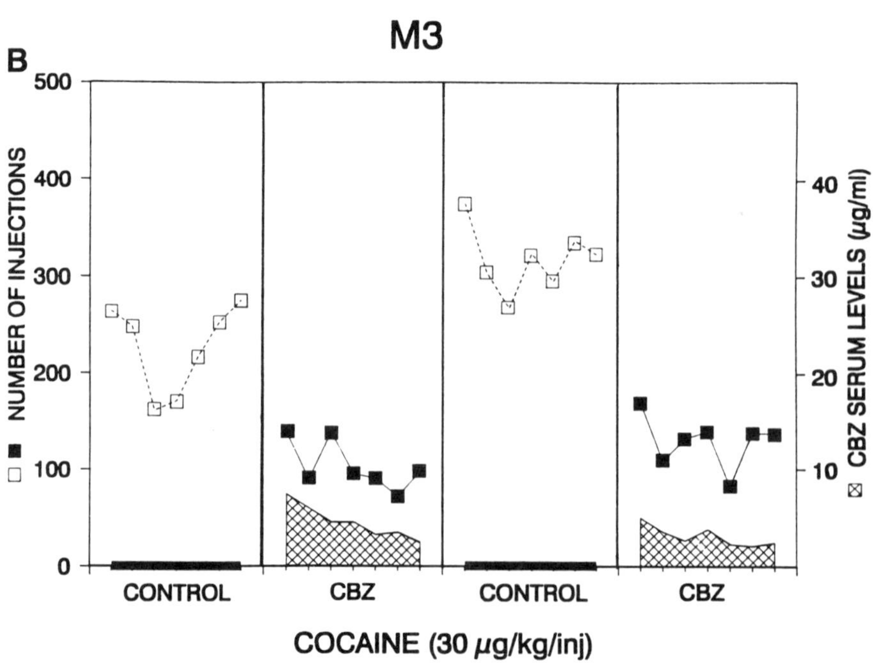
B
M3
500
400
300
200
100
0
NUMBER OF INJECTIONS
40
30
20
10
CBZ SERUM LEVELS (μg/ml)
CONTROL
CBZ
CONTROL
CBZ
COCAINE (30 μg/kg/inj)

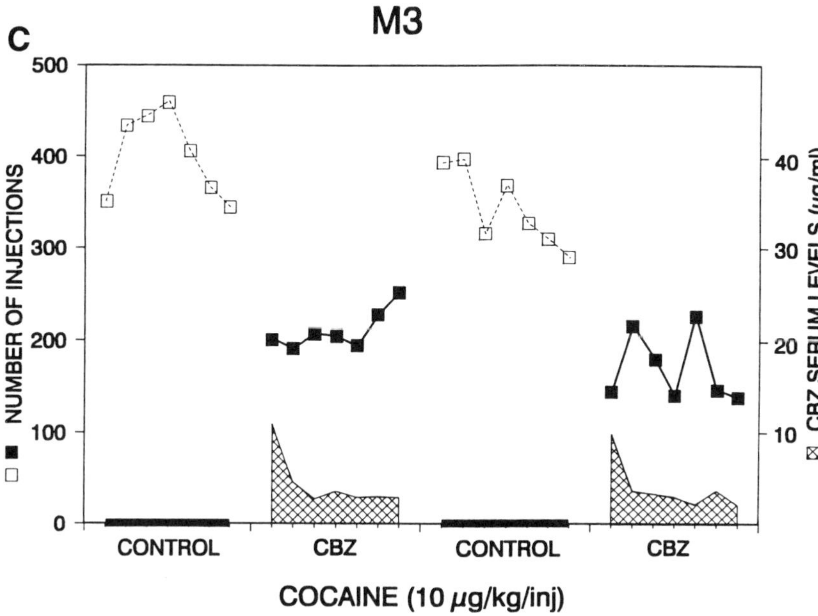

Fig. 8. Carbamazepine more effectively decreases cocaine self-administration in rhesus monkeys at lower cocaine doses, associated with higher rates of responding. Figures 8**A, B,** and **C** illustrate the number of cocaine injections self-administered each day by a monkey on (solid squares) and off (open squares) carbamazepine treatment. The doses of cocaine illustrated are **(A)** 100, **(B)** 30, and **(C)** 10 µg/kg/injection. Carbamazepine blood levels are shown on the same graphs (crosshatched), and these fall within the low therapeutic range for patients.

carbamazepine blood levels were falling, low, or nonexistent. Further study would be required to determine the reasons for these apparent discrepancies in carbamazepine's safety. In any event, similar to our primate study, carbamazepine had minimal effects on groups of rats with lower baseline rates of cocaine self-administration and more marked effects on higher rates of self-administration.

Sharpe et al.[31] reported nonspecific inhibitory effects of carbamazepine on both cocaine self-administration and on food intake in rats at the most recent CPDD meeting. It is noteworthy that in their study they used repeated intermittent administration of carbamazepine (15 mg/kg, ip). Although this dose is highly effective in inhibiting completed amygdala-kindled seizures, as we noted earlier, it is without effect on cocaine-kindled seizure evolution or cocaine seizure-associated lethality. Moreover, carbamazepine can be sedating when given ip at that dose, in contrast to when it is given in the diet where behavioral sedation is not observed. Thus, we do not believe that the results of that study suggesting that carbamazepine would affect food intake would extrapolate to those achieved with oral administration in the rhesus monkeys or would apply to more chronic oral administration in humans where impact on food intake has not been an issue.

Mechanisms of Carbamazepine Relevant to Inhibition of Cocaine and Self-Administration

Carbamazepine is a complex drug with multiple effects on neurotransmitter, neuropeptide, and second messenger systems in brain.[14–16] We have begun a systematic attempt to dissect possible mechanisms involved in its ability to block cocaine-kindled seizures based on the notion (explicated earlier) that effects that require chronic administration also may be pertinent to the psychotropic effects of the drug. Such a dissection may also yield information pertinent to carbamazepine's action on cocaine self-administration.

We had previously demonstrated that the acute anticonvulsant effects of carbamazepine on amygdala-kindled seizures were closely related to its effects on peripheral-type benzodiazepine receptors.[32,33] The anticonvulsant effects of carbamazepine are blocked by the peripheral-type ligand Ro5-4864, but are not blocked by the central-type benzodiazepine antagonist RO-15-1788. This is the converse of the effects on diazepam, where the central antagonist RO-15-1788 effectively reverses diazepam's anticonvulsant effect, but Ro5-4864 is ineffective. However, we do not believe it likely that peripheral-type benzodiazepine receptors are involved in the chronic effects of carbamazepine on local-anesthetic-kindled seizures. The two types of seizures show different responses to carbamazepine based on acute vs chronic administration and as a function of stage of seizure development (development vs completed). Thus, we have begun to explore other possible candidate systems that might be involved in the chronic anticonvulsant effects of carbamazepine on cocaine-kindled seizures.

Utilizing this paradigm, we have identified several neurotransmitter and neuropeptide systems that are not critical to carbamazepine's chronic actions in inhibiting local-anesthetic-kindled seizures. These data are summarized in Table 2. For example, although the α_2 antagonist yohimbine blocks

Table 2
Pharmacological Blockade of Carbamazepine's Effects on Cocaine Seizures

System	Drug	Dose	Effect on cocaine kindling	Effect on CBZ's anticonvulsant actions
α_2 antagonism	Yohimbine	5 mg/kg	Potentiates	None*
Serotonin depletion	PCPA	300 mg/kg × 3 d prior to cocaine, then q-wkly during kindling	None	None
Cholinergic:				
blockade	Atropine	20 mg/kg	Attenuates	Potentiates
potentiation	Physostigmine	0.5 mg/kg	None	None
Somatostatin depletion	Cysteamine	200 mg/kg		
		4 h	Potentiates	?
		24 h	Potentitates	?
Adenosine upregulation	Caffeine preRx:			
	Diet (600 mg/kg food) × 3 wk		Attenuates	?
	Caffeine preRx + cotreatment			
	Diet × 3 wk + 20 mg/kg		None	?
p-Type Benzo-diazepine receptors				
Antagonism	PK11195**	30 mg/kg	None (lidocaine)	?
Agonism	RO5-4864*	10 mg/kg	Potentiates	None
CRH	5, 10, 100 μg (icv)		Potentiates	
	10, 100 μg (icv)			Blocks
Tricyclic anti-depressant	DMI	10 mg/kg 2X d 5 d preRx + 10 mg/kg during K	Potentiates	?

*None on CBZ inhibition of cocaine kindling, but will inhibit CBZ effects on amygdala kindling.
**PK11195 was given acutely; drug should be restudied (like CBZ) with chronic administration.

the acute anticonvulsant effects of carbamazepine on amygdala-kindled seizures, it does not block carbamazepine's effects on cocaine-kindled seizures suggesting, that α_2 mechanisms are not critical. A similar lack of blockade of carbamazepine's anticonvulsant effects was found for PCPA and atropine, suggesting that serotonergic and cholinergic systems are also not crucial to carbamazepine's effects on cocaine-kindled seizures (Weiss et al., 1990,1991, unpublished observations). The somatostatin-depleting agent cysteamine potentiated cocaine-kindled seizures, suggesting that carbamazepine's ability to decrease somatostatin levels is not responsible for its chronic anticonvulsant actions. In contrast, icv administration of corticotropin-releasing hormone (CRH) does block the anticonvulsant effects of carbamazepine on cocaine-kindled seizures, although only at doses that given by themselves potentiate cocaine-kindled seizure development and lethality *(34)*. Thus, it remains to be demonstrated whether CRH is involved in carbamazepine's mechanism of action on this seizure type.

The CRH system is of considerable interest in relation to psychotropic and anticonvulsant effects. Abnormalities in CRH release and cortisol regulation have been demonstrated in affective disorders and CRH has been shown to produce seizures in rats following icv administration. CRH release in hypothalamic explants can be induced by local anesthetics and this effect is blocked by carbamazepine *(35)*. Carbamazepine also inhibits local-anesthetic-induced release of ACTH and cortisol *(36)*. CRH is also implicated in behavioral sensitization to amphetamine and cross-sensitization to stress *(37,38)*, although it does not appear critical for context-dependent cocaine sensitization (Weiss et al., unpublished observations). Adrenalectomy has been reported to block behavioral sensitization following repeated amphetamine administration or restraint stress. Most recently, Piazza et al. *(39)* reported that animals with greater corticosterone levels showed greater activation by amphetamine and an increased predisposition to amphetamine self-administration. Thus, on a variety of levels the CRH system appears to be involved in mechanisms of stress, sensitization, seizure evolution, and psychopathology.

Thus, it is possible that the complex effects of carbamazepine, not only on CRH release,[35] but other aspects of the hypothalamic-pituitary-adrenal axis,[40–42] could be important to its effects on cocaine-kindling evolution, if not on self-administration. Further work is required to elucidate the possible mechanisms involved in the blockade by carbamazepine of cocaine self-administration and to substantiate the specificity of this effect.

Although such studies may be crucial to understanding the mechanisms of action of carbamazepine on kindled seizure evolution and on self-administration, it appears that only prospective, double-blind, controlled clinical studies will adequately elucidate whether this drug will be useful in the treatment of various aspects of cocaine abuse disorders.

Clinical Studies of Carbamazepine in Cocaine Abusers

Halikas, based on our preclinical data with cocaine kindling, postulated that carbamazepine might be effective in cocaine abuse disorders through its kindling-like inhibition properties. He performed an open clinical trial, finding that low doses of carbamazepine administered to cocaine and heroin abusers resulted in a subgroup of patients who markedly decreased their cocaine intake while taking carbamazepine on a regular basis.[43] Another subgroup of patients who took the drug more sporadically showed partial effects, and the third group that stopped taking the drug showed no change in their cocaine intake, as measured by the number of urines testing positive for cocaine before and during the study.

These promising initial open observations have led to a series of double-blind, controlled clinical trials. The first such trial was completed by Halikas' group and suggested some efficacy of the carbamazepine (if blood levels were >4 µg/mL) in decreasing the number of positive cocaine urines in an unmotivated group of subjects.[44] The data from further controlled studies are eagerly awaited from other groups, including those in Philadelphia[45] and Baltimore (Gorelick).

Hatsukami et al.[9] reported a lack of effect of carbamazepine on acute subjective responses to smoked cocaine base in human cocaine users. These data are in accord with the psychomotor stimulant data in animals discussed earlier, as well as the data of Meyendorff et al.[8] on the inability of carbamazepine to block methylphenidate-induced euphoria. In the study of Hatsukami, significantly higher heart rate, diastolic blood pressure, and blood pressure/heart rate product were observed following carbamazepine administration compared with placebo in subjects who smoked a 40-mg dose of cocaine. Noradrenergic effects of carbamazepine may be responsible for this observation. The α_2 agonist clonidine, when administered directly into brain, has been shown to increase blood pressure,[46] and carbamazepine has been shown to antagonize this effect.[47] These and other data suggest that carbamazepine could possess α_2 antagonist properties or other mechanisms sufficient to interfere with noradrenergic regulation of blood pressure.

The data on carbamazepine's effects on noradrenergic mechanisms are complex, and they appear to differ across seizure type as well. For example, we have found that yohimbine reverses the anticonvulsant effects of carbamazepine on amygdala-kindled seizures, whereas opposite effects have been reported on electroconvulsive seizures. In the latter, yohimbine increases the seizure threshold and potentiates carbamazepine's effects,[48] whereas clonidine acts in the opposite fashion.[49] Carbamazepine acutely increases firing of the locus coeruleus by unknown mechanisms,[50,51] and yet is also associated with decreases in noradrenergic turnover.[52] Thus, carbamazepine may have interactions with acute cocaine injections that could be relevant to autonomic and blood pressure regulation.[9] These may differ from other effects of cocaine where carbamazepine counters the effects of cocaine on kindled seizure evolution and self-administration.

We are also currently exploring the utility of carbamazepine administration in blocking the subjective and physiological effects of procaine,[53] another local anesthetic without prominent psychomotor stimulant properties. It is possible that the shared ability of carbamazepine and local anesthetics to interact with the batrachotoxin-sensitive type II sodium channels[54,55] could be implicated in the effects of the drug on cocaine kindling and self-administration. However, a wide variety of other mechanisms, reviewed elsewhere,[14–16] remain as candidate systems for carbamazepine's effects on cocaine kindling, as well as its anticonvulsant and psychotropic properties. Thus, much work remains to be done in order to elucidate the precise mechanisms of this agent involved with different aspects of its clinical profile.

Clinical Implications and Conclusion

Although the precise mechanisms of action of carbamazepine remain to be elucidated, the results of the clinical studies of the efficacy of carbamazepine in cocaine abuse disorders are eagerly awaited. Should these be positive, at least in some aspects, carbamazepine holds promise in the treatment of cocaine abuse disorders for a variety of ancillary reasons. There is wide experience in its use in the treatment of paroxysmal pain disorders, seizure disorders, and now in the acute and prophylactic treatment of mood disorders.[56] In addition, carbamazepine has been reported to have clinical utility in the treatment of disorders of aggression such as episodic dyscontrol,[57] borderline personality disorder,[58] and others.[13,59] Finally, no abuse potential for carbamazepine has been reported in the over 20 yr of its use in epileptic syndromes.

Thus, carbamazepine's diverse clinical profile in some ways appears ideally suited for use in a cocaine-addicted population. Carbamazepine has been widely used in Europe and more recently in some controlled clinical trials in the United States as a substitute for benzodiazepines in alcohol withdrawal syndromes and more extended postwithdrawal treatment.[60–63] This has been of great potential utility, since benzodiazepines, although effective in treating anxiety disorders, have a high abuse potential in those with alcohol addiction problems and in polysubstance abusers. Thus, to the extent that cocaine use may be a comorbid condition in patients with affective disorders, alcohol abuse problems, and polysubstance abuse, carbamazepine might have a role in also targeting the symptoms of these disorders or, at least, not presenting an additional abuse liability.

To the extent that carbamazepine's ability to block cocaine-kindled seizure evolution in the rat is paralleled by a similar effect in humans (independent of its ability to inhibit self-administration), carbamazepine might be useful in the long-term treatment of cocaine abusers, with the idea that it could ameliorate some of the side effects associated with repeated cocaine administration. These might include inhibition of seizure development and even panic attacks. Elsewhere, we have discussed how repeated cocaine administration might be associated with a kindling-like evolution of panic attacks, ultimately leading to the spontaneous variety.[64,65] To the extent that carbamazepine blocks the local-anesthetic kindling process, which might be mediating panic attack evolution, we would predict that it might also inhibit panic attacks from developing.

Although the preclinical data are promising, clinical studies in cocaine users will form the critical basis for the potential utility of carbamazepine in treatment of cocaine abuse disorders. Further data from these studies will determine whether this drug will be useful in the treatment of this difficult syndrome, and investigation into the mechanism of action of carbamazepine may lead to other newer and more targeted treatment strategies as well.

Acknowledgment

The authors express their appreciation to NIDA for supplementary funds for support of this research.

References

[1]R. M. Post (1981) Lidocaine kindled limbic seizures: behavioral implications, in *Kindling 2*. J. A. Wada, ed. Raven, New York, pp. 149–160.

[2]R. M. Post, C. Kennedy, M. Shinohara, K. Squillace, M. Miyaoka, S. Suda, D. H. Ingvar, and L. Sokoloff (1984) Metabolic and behavioral consequences of lidocaine-kindled seizures. *Brain Res.* **324,** 295–303.

[3]R. M. Post, R. T. Kopanda, A. Lee (1975) Progressive behavioral changes during chronic lidocaine administration: relationship to kindling. *Life Sci.* **17,** 943–950.

[4]S. R. B. Weiss, M. Costello, R. Woodward, D. J. Nutt, and R. M. Post (1987) Chronic carbamazepine inhibits the development of cocaine-kindled seizures. *Soc. Neurosci. Abstracts* **13,** 950.

[5]S. R. B. Weiss, R. M. Post, M. Costello, Nutt D, S. Tandeciarz, J. Nierenberg, R. Lewis, and M. Clark (1989) Carbamazepine prevents cocaine-kindled seizures and lethality but does not interfere with behavioral sensitization. *Abstracts, American College of Neuropsychopharmacology* 236.

[6]S. R. B. Weiss, R. M. Post, F. Szele, R. Woodward, and J. Nierenberg (1989) Chronic carbamazepine inhibits the development of local anesthetic seizures kindled by cocaine and lidocaine. *Brain Res.* **497,** 72–79.

[7]S. R. B. Weiss, Post M, M. Costello, D. J. Nutt, and S. Tandeciarz (1990) Carbamazepine retards the development of cocaine-kindled seizures but not sensitization to cocaine's effects on hyperactivity and stereotypy. *Neuropsychopharmacology* **3,** 273–281.

[8]E. Meyendorff, B. Lerer, N. C. Moore, J. Bow, and S. Gershon (1985) Methylphenidate infusion in euthymic bipolars: effect of carbamazepine pretreatment. *Psychiatry* Res. **16,** 303.

[9]D. Hatsukami, R. Keenan, J. Halikas, P. R. Pentel, and L. H. Brauer (1991) Effects of carbamazepine on acute responses to smoked cocaine-base in human cocaine users. *Psychopharmacology* **104**, 120–124.

[10]T. Aigner, S. R. B. Weiss, and R. M. Post (1990) Carbamazepine attenuates i.v. cocaine self-administration in rhesus monkeys. *Abstracts, ACNP* 181.

[11]P. J. Marangos, S. R. B. Weiss, P. Montgomery, J. Patel, P. K. Narang, A. Cappabianca, and R. M. Post (1985) Chronic carbamazepine treatment increases brain adenosine receptors. *Epilepsia* **26,** 493–498.

[12]R. M. Post, S. R. B. Weiss, F. Szele, and R. Woodward (1986) Differential anticonvulsant effects of carbamazepine as a function of stage and type of kindling. *Soc. Neurosci. Abstracts* **12,** 1375.

[13]R. M. Post, L. L. Altshuler, T. Ketter, K. Denicoff, and S. R. B. Weiss (1991) Antiepileptic drugs in affective illness: Clinical and theoretical implications, in *Advances in Neurology, vol. 55, Neurobehavioral Problems in Epilepsy.* D. B. Smith, D. M. Treiman, and M. R. Trimble, eds. Raven, New York, pp. 239–277.

[14]R. M. Post, S. R. B. Weiss, and D.-M. Chuang (1992) Mechanisms of action of anticonvulsants in affective disorders: Comparisons with lithium. *J. Clin. Psychopharmacol.* **12,** 235–355.

[15]R. M. Post (1987) Mechanisms of action of carbamazepine and related anticonvulsants in affective illness, in *Psychopharmacology: A Generation of Progress.* H. Meltzer and W. E. Bunney Jr., eds. Raven, New York, pp. 567–576.

[16]R. M. Post (1988) Time course of clinical effects of carbamazepine: implications for mechanisms of action. *J. Clin. Psychiatry* **49,** 35–46.

[17]S. R. B. Weiss and R. M. Post (1987) Carbamazepine and carbamazepine-10,11–epoxide inhibit amygdala kindled seizures in the rat but do not block their development. *Clin. Neuropharmacol.* **10,** 272–279.

[18]W. P. Koella, P. Levin, and V. Baltzer (1976) The pharmacology of carbamazepine and some other anti-epileptic drugs, in *Epileptic Seizures—Behavior—Pain.* Birkmayer W, ed. Hans Huber, Bern, pp. 32–50.

[19]S. R. B. Weiss, R. M. Post, A. Pert, R. Woodward, and D. Murman (1989) Context-dependent cocaine sensitization: Differential effect of haloperidol on development versus expression. *Pharmacol. Biochem. Behav.* **34,** 655–661.

[20]R. M. Post, S. R. B. Weiss, and A. Pert (1984) Differential effects of carbamazepine and lithium on sensitization and kindling. *Prog. Neuropsychopharmacol. Biol. Psychiatry* **8,** 425–434.

[21]P. H. Kelly and S. D. Iversen (1976) Selective 60HDA-induced destruction of mesolimbic dopamine neurons: abolition of psychostimulant-induced locomotor activity in rats. *Eur. J Pharmacol.* **40,** 45–56.

[22]D. C. S. Roberts, G. F. Koob, P. Klanoff, and H. C. Fibiger (1980) Extinction and recovery of cocaine self-administration following 6–hydroxydopamine lesions of the nucleus accumbens. *Pharmacol. Biochem. Behav.* **12,** 781–787.

[23]R. M. Post, S. R. B. Weiss, and A. Pert (1988) Cocaine-induced behavioral sensitization and kindling: implications for the emergence of psychopathology and seizures, in *Mesocorticolimbic Dopamine System.* P. W. Kalivas and C. B. Nemeroff, eds. New York Academy of Science, New York, pp. 292–308.

[24]R. M. Post, S. R. B. Weiss, and A. Pert (1991) Animal models of mania, in *The Mesolimbic Dopamine System: From Motivation to Action.* P. Willner and J. Scheel-Kruger, eds. Wiley, Chichester, England, pp. 443–472.

[25]R. M. Post and S. R. B. Weiss (1988) Psychomotor stimulant versus local anesthetic effects of cocaine: role of behavioral sensitization and kindling, in *Mechanisms of Cocaine Abuse and Toxicity* (NIDA Research Monograph 88). US Government Printing Office, Washington, DC, pp. 217–238.

[26]D. C. S. Roberts, M. E. Corcoran, and H. C. Fibiger (1977) On the rate of ascending catecholaminergic systems in iv self-administration of cocaine. *Pharmacol. Biochem. Behav.* **6,** 615–620.

[27]K. A. Zito, G. Vickers, and D. C. Roberts (1985) Disruption of cocaine and

heroin self-administration following kainic acid lesions of the nucleus accumbens. *Pharmacol. Biochem. Behav.* **23,** 1029–1036.

[28]G. F. Koob (1988) Separate neurochemical substrates for cocaine and heroin reinforcement, in *Quantitative Analyses of Behavior: Biological Determinants of Reinforcement.* M. L. Commons, R. M. Church, J. R. Stellar, and A. R. Wagner, eds. Erlbaum, Hillsdale, NJ, pp. 139–156.

[29]H. O. Pettit, A. Ettenberg, F. E. Bloom, and G. F. Koob (1984) Destruction of dopamine in the nucleus accumbens selectively attenuates cocaine but not heroin self-administration in rats. *Psychopharmacology* **84,** 167–173.

[30]M. E. Carroll, S. T. Lac, M. Asencio, J. A. Halikas, and R. Kragh (1990) Effects of carbamazepine on self-administration of intravenously delivered cocaine in rats. *Pharmacol. Biochem. Behav.* **37,** 551–556.

[31]L. G. Sharpe, F. J. Nouvet, J. L. Katz, and J. H. Jaffe. Nonspecific effects of carbamazepine on cocaine self-administration in rats. Abstracts, CPDD 1.

[32]S. R. B. Weiss, R. M. Post, J. Patel, and P. J. Marangos (1985) Differential mediation of the anticonvulsant effects of carbamazepine and diazepam. *Life Sci..* **36,** 2413–2419.

[33]S. R. B. Weiss, R. M. Post, P. J. Marangos, and J. Patel (1986) Peripheral-type benzodiazepines: behavioral effects and interactions with the anticonvulant effects of carbamazepine, in *Kindling III.* J. Wada, ed. Raven, New York, pp. 375–392.

[34]S. R. B. Weiss, J. Nierenberg, R. Lewis, and R. M. Post (1992) Corticotropin-releasing hormone: Potentiation of cocaine kindled seizures and lethality. *Epilepsia* in press.

[35]A. E. Calogero, W. T. Gallucci, M. A. Kling, G. P. Chrousos, and P. W. Gold (1989) Cocaine stimulates rat hypothalamic corticotropin-releasing hormone secretion in vitro. *Brain Res.* **505,** 7–11.

[36]A. E. Calogero, M. A. Kling, W. T. Gallucci, C. Saoutis, R. M. Post, G. P. Chrousos, and P. W. Gold (1987) Local anaesthetics procaine and lidocaine stimulate corticotropin releasing hormone secretion in vitro: clinical implications. *Soc. Neurosci. Abstracts* **13,** 1163 Abs. #319.2.

[37]B. J. Cole, M. Cador, L. Stinus, J. Rivier, W. Vale, G. F. Koob, and M. Le Moal (1990) Central administration of a CRF antagonist blocks the development of stress-induced behavioral sensitization. *Brain Res.* **512,** 343–346.

[38]M. Cador, B. J. Cole, L. Stinus, G. F. Koob, and M. Le Moal (1991) Endogenous CRF: Role in stress- and amphetamine-induced behavioral sensitization 1. *NY Acad. Sci.* Abstract 1.

[39]P. V. Piazza, S. Maccari, J.-M. Deminiere, M. Le Moal, P. Mormede, and H. Simon (1991) Corticosterone levels determine individual vulnerability to amphetamine self-administration. *Proc. Natl. Acad. Sci. USA* **88,** 2088–2092.

[40]D. R. Rubinow, R. M. Post, and P. W. Gold (1984) Neuroendocrine and peptide effects of carbamazepine: clinical and theoretical implications. *Psychopharmacol. Bull.* **20,** 590–594.

[41]D. R. Rubinow, R. M. Post, P. W. Gold, J. C. Ballenger, and E. A. Wolff (1984) The relationship between cortisol and clinical phenomenology of affective illness, in *Neurobiology of Mood Disorders*. R. M. Post and J. C. Ballenger, eds. Williams and Wilkins, Baltimore, MD, pp. 271–289.

[42]D. R. Rubinow, R. M. Post, P. W. Gold, and S. Reichlin (1985) Effects of carbamazepine on cerebrospinal fluid somatostatin. *Psychopharmacology* **85,** 210–214.

[43]J. Halikas, K. Kemp, K. Kuhn, G. Carlson, and F. Crea (1989) Carbamazepine for cocaine addiction? [letter]. *Lancet* **1,** 623–624.

[44]J. A. Halikas, R. D. Crosby, G. A. Carlson, F. Crea, N. M. Graves, and L. D. Bowers (1990) Double-blind cocaine reduction in unmotivated crack users: Carbamazepine versus placebo in a short term crossover design. *Abstracts, ACNP* 217.

[45]C. P. O'Brien, A. R. Childress, I. O. Arndt, A. T. McLellan, G. E. Woody, and I. Maany (1988) Pharmacological and behavioral treatments of cocaine dependence: controlled studies. *J. Clin. Psychiatry* **49,** 17–22.

[46]H. Kawasaki, S. Nakamura, and K. Takasaki (1991) Somatostatin inhibits the centrally mediated hypertensive response to clonidine in freely moving rats. *Neurosci. Lett.* **123,** 232–235.

[47]R. Mosqueda-Garcia, J. A. Oates, M. Appalsamy, and D. Robertson (1991) Administration of carbamazepine in the nucleus of the solitary tract inhibits the antihypertensive effect of clonidine. *Eur. J Pharmacol.* **197,** 213–216.

[48]W. Fischer and M. Muller (1988) Pharmacological modulation of central monoaminergic systems and influence on the anticonvulsant effectiveness of standard antiepileptics in maximal electroshock seizure. *Biomed. Biochim. Acta* **47,** 631–645.

[49]V. Crunelli, L. Cervo, and R. Samanin (1981) Evidence for a preferential role of central noradrenergic neurons in electrically induced convulsions and activity of various anticonvulsants in the rat, in *Neurotransmitters, Seizures and Epilepsy*. P. L. Morselli, K. G. Lloyd, and W. Loscher, eds. Raven, New York, pp. 195–202.

[50]H. R. Olpe and R. Jones (1983) The action of anticonvulsant drugs on the firing of locus coeruleus neurons: selective, activating effect of carbamazepine. *Eur. J Pharmacol.* **91,** 107–110.

[51]H. R. Olpe (1991) Mechanism of action of antiepileptic drugs with special reference to carbamazepine. *Abstracts, World Congress Biol. Psychiatry* **29,** 185.

[52]L. Maitre, V. Baltzer, and C. Mondadori (1984) Psychopharmacological and behavioural effects of anti-epileptic drugs in animals, in *Anticonvulsants in Affective Disorders*. H. M. Emrich, T. Okuma, and M. Muller, eds. Excerpta Medica, Amsterdam, pp. 3–13.

[53]C. H. Kellner, R. M. Post, F. Putnam, R. W. Cowdry, D. Gardner, M. A. Kling, M. D. Minichiello, J. R. Trettau, and R. Coppola (1987) IV procaine as a probe of limbic system activity in psychiatric patients and normal controls. *Biol. Psychiatry* **22,** 1107–1126.

[54]M. Willow and W. A Catterall (1982) Inhibition of binding of [^{3}H] batrachotoxinin A 20-alpha-benzoate to sodium channels by the anticonvulsant drugs diphenylhydantoin and carbamazepine. *Mol. Pharmacol.* **22**, 627–635.

[55]M. J. McLean and R. L. Macdonald (1986) Carbamazepine and 10,11-epoxycarbamazepine produce use- and voltage-dependent limitation of rapidly firing action potentials of mouse central neurons in cell culture. *J. Pharmacol. Exp. Ther.* **238**, 727–738.

[56]R. M. Post (1990) Alternatives to lithium for bipolar affective illness, in *Review of Psychiatry, vol. 9.* A. Tasman, S. M. Goldfinger, and C. A. Kaufmann, eds. American Psychiatric Press, Washington, DC, pp. 170–202.

[57]J. A. Mattes (1984) Carbamazepine for uncontrolled rage outbursts. *Lancet* **2**, 1164–1165.

[58]R. W. Cowdry and D. L. Gardner (1988) Pharmacotherapy of borderline personality disorder. *Arch. Gen. Psychiatry* **111**, 119.

[59]P. P. Roy-Byrne, T. W. Uhde, and R. M. Post (1984) Carbamazepine for aggression, schizophrenia, and nonaffective syndromes. *Int. Drug Ther. Newslett.* **19**, 9–12.

[60]J. C. Ballenger and R. M. Post (1984) Carbamazepine in alcohol withdrawal syndromes and schizophrenic psychoses. *Psychopharmacol. Bull.* **20**, 572–584.

[61]J. C. Ballenger and R. M. Post (1989) Addictive behavior and kindling: relationship to alcohol withdrawal and cocaine, in *The Clinical Relevance of Kindling*. M. Trimble and T. G. Bolwig, eds. Wiley, West Essex, England, pp. 231–258.

[62]R. Malcolm, J. C. Ballenger, E. T. Sturgis, and R. Anton (1989) Double-blind controlled trial comparing carbamazepine to oxazepam treatment of alcohol withdrawal. *Am. J. Psychiatry* **146**, 617–621.

[63]C. H. Stuppaeck, C. Barnas, K. Hackenberg, C. H. Miller, and W. W. Fleischhacker (1990) Carbamazepine monotherapy in the treatment of alcohol withdrawal. *Intern. Clin. Psychopharmacol.* **5**, 273–278.

[64]R. M. Post, S. R. B. Weiss, A. Pert, and T. W. Uhde (1987) Chronic cocaine administration: sensitization and kindling effects, in *Cocaine: Clinical and Biobehavioral Aspects.* A. Raskin, and S. Fisher, eds. Oxford University Press, New York, pp. 109–173.

[65]R. M. Post, S. R. B. Weiss, T. W. Uhde, M. Clark, and J. B. Rosen (1992) Preclinical neuroscience advances pertinent to panic disorder: Implications of cocaine kindling, induction of the proto-oncogene c-fos, and contingent tolerance, in *Biology of Anxiety Disorders: Recent Developments.* R. Hoehn-Saric, ed. American Psychiatric Press, Washington, DC, in press.

Relapse Prevention for the Cocaine and Crack Dependent

An Essential Treatment Component

Barbara C. Wallace

Introduction

The cocaine and crack epidemic of the 1980s challenged the field of chemical dependency treatment to refine its methods and modalities. Among the various changes implemented, the emphasis on relapse prevention emerges as the most significant innovation in the overall field of chemical dependence, and it is absolutely critical in treating the cocaine and crack dependent. As we negotiate chemical dependency treatment in the 1990s, we are fortunate in finding few new initiates of crack cocaine smoking. However, a cohort of crack cocaine smokers will continue to seek treatment in the 1990s, while the continued use of intranasal and intravenous cocaine is also likely to create a substantial subset of chemically dependent admissions who require efficacious treatment. Such treatment must include relapse prevention as an essential component. This chapter presents relevant historical background, reviews professionals'

From: *Drug and Alcohol Abuse Reviews, Vol. 4: Drug Abuse Treatment*
Ed: R. R. Watson ©1992 The Humana Press Inc.

views on relapse, provides a biopsychosocial approach to relapse, summarizes pertinent research, describes exemplary models of relapse prevention, and discusses future directions in relapse prevention.

A Historical Perspective on Relapse

The contemporary study of the problem of relapse among the cocaine and crack dependent finds its roots in the work of Hunt et al.,[1] whose inverted J-shape curve depicts how about two-thirds of cigaret smokers, alcoholics, and heroin addicts experienced a relapse within the first 90 d following treatment. In search of the apparent common mechanism underlying relapse across a variety of addictive substances, Cummings et al.[2] analyzed initial relapse episodes among problem drinkers, cigaret smokers, heroin addicts, overeaters, and compulsive gamblers. These researchers found that major determinants of relapse episodes included negative emotional states (35%), interpersonal conflict (16%), and social pressure (20%). Building on these research findings, Marlatt and Gordon[3] utilized a cognitive–behavioral framework in establishing the foundation on which the contemporary study of relapse rests. The work of Marlatt and Gordon[3] has been the starting point of virtually all attempts to initiate research into the determinants of relapse for various addictions and for designing relapse prevention programs.

Key concepts taken from Marlatt's seminal body of work include the following: the concept of the abstinence violation effect (AVE); the notion of apparently irrelevant decisions (AIDS); the distinction between a slip or lapse and a full-blown relapse; the importance of lifestyle modification; the importance of relapse as a learning experience; the task of engaging in a microanalysis of the relapse episode so that determinants of that relapse can be identified and the relapse episode utilized as an opportunity for learning; and, the idea that we must go beyond the disease model notion of internal causation so we can teach clients to appreciate external determinants of relapse to which they can respond by executing alternative behaviors, thereby avoiding a relapse.[3] Marlatt and Gordon[3] also encourage the use of metaphor that proves to be especially effective in bypassing defenses of denial and resistance commonly found in the addict.[4]

Most treatment professionals who had to face the challenging cocaine and crack population of the 1980s turned to this body of work and followed Marlatt's leadership as they struggled to prolong the period of abstinence and reduce the frequency of slips and relapses within this population. However, their professional views and the clinical technique they deployed to manage the high relapse potential associated with the cocaine and crack population also evolved out of the raw data of observation—obtained while on the front-line treating addicts during the height of the 1980s cocaine and crack epidemic.

Professionals' Views on Relapse

A review and analysis of numerous professionals' writings on relapse in the cocaine and crack dependent population[5–15] suggests several important points. First and foremost, professionals view relapse as a process that occurs over a period of time, preceding and including the exact moment when a person who has attempted abstinence from a chemical for some period of time returns to chemical use. Secondly, relapse involves multiple determinants that frequently act in concert in producing a relapse episode. Thirdly, evidence of multiple determinants acting in concert to produce a relapse episode is also suggested in clinicians' selection of a variety of treatment interventions derived from different theoretical schools of thought. The result being that diverse clinicians tend to utilize a multifaceted clinical technique combining education, cognitive–behavioral interventions, elements of a psychodynamic technique, and use of metaphorical forms of communication.

These clinicians' refinement of a multifaceted clinical technique arose from their observation of several factors that lead to relapse in the cocaine and crack dependent population treated in inpatient and outpatient settings:

1. Drug craving;
2. Recurrent selective recall of cocaine euphoria;
3. The provocative power of drug associated environmental cues;
4. Processes of denial and addictive thinking that permit patients setting themselves up;
5. Myths/delusions of being able to sell, use, or be around cocaine or other drugs; and
6. Recurrent painful affect states previously self-medicated with cocaine.

Clinicians' use of education and cognitive interventions addresses several of these factors involving clients' possession of false beliefs and dangerous cognitions likely to lead to relapse. The use of metaphorical forms of communication—such as the telling of stories and actual sharing of metaphors—both conveys critical education and serves to bypass clients' defenses. Elements of a psychodynamic technique address denial, defensive functioning, and management of painful affect states. Behavioral interventions are relied on to address the evocative power of classically conditioned stimuli, which may readily bring about a conditioned response of craving or drug use.

Thus, a summary and analysis of numerous front-line treatment professionals' views further builds on the seminal work of Marlatt and Gordon.[3] In effect, these professionals have assisted in the further evolution of the contemporary study of relapse in the cocaine and crack dependent population. As we have seen, professionals' views on the process and determinants of relapse cannot be separated from their refinement and implementation of a multifaceted clinical technique that combines educational, psychodynamic, cognitive–behavioral, and metaphorical interventions.

A Biopsychosocial Model of Addiction and Relapse Prevention

Biopsychosocial models of addiction are emerging as the only acceptable standard in the field,[16–18] permitting professionals to categorize their observations of the relapse process. A biopsychosocial model of cocaine and crack dependence follows, which elucidates the need to reduce the chances of relapse by addressing biological, psychological, and social–environmental dimensions of addiction.

The Biological Domain and Relapse Prevention

Since cocaine is the most reinforcing or most addicting drug—as suggested in animal laboratory studies—and crack is the most addictive form of cocaine,[19] the importance of a biological understanding of the actions of cocaine and crack emerges as paramount. In fact, understanding of the biological actions of cocaine, cocaine's pharmacology, and a cocaine withdrawal syndrome[20] is essential if we are to achieve empathy for the client's predicament. We easily fail in treating the cocaine and crack dependent when we do not possess empathy. The only way to achieve empathy at the very start is to possess knowledge of cocaine and crack's biological actions.

How can one empathize with a pregnant crack addict who arrives at the emergency room in labor straight from a crack house, and whose primary concern after delivery of a prenatally crack-exposed infant is leaving the hospital to secure yet another "hit" of crack? Or, how can we empathize with an upper middle-class male client who emphasizes that he free-bases (i.e., prepares his own smokeable form of the cocaine alkaloid, which can be called free-base instead of crack to avoid the stigma attached to crack smokers) as he explains how he sold company secrets for drug money, while losing his job, wife, children, family home, and thousands in savings because of his addiction? Meanwhile, both the female and male crack smoker test positive for venereal disease, have passed it on to fetus and spouse, and even placed themselves and others at risk for HIV infection because of sexual promiscuity associated with their crack/cocaine use. It is the easiest thing in the world to hate and despise such clients. Thus, the only way one can even begin to achieve empathy with such severely dependent crack or cocaine clients is to understand the biological basis of addiction. At the same time, we can begin to grasp the urgency of reducing the chances of relapse by addressing factors falling under the biological domain.

Professionals routinely observe clients such as those painted in the two prototypical caricatures. They enter treatment and report several attempts to stop on their own—such as when the pregnancy was first discovered or the supervisor at work gave the first warning. Within assessments, professionals hear a brief relapse history embedded in such tales. These histories of relapse and failed attempts to stop on their own reveal how clients in withdrawal from cocaine/crack resume drug use after several hours or several days since last cocaine/crack use because of intense brain-driven cravings.[20] Others have referred to this same biologically based phenomenon as involving intense neurochemically based cravings,[19] which lead to resumption of cocaine/crack use.

Use of the term relapse after a 2- or 3-d period of attempted abstinence may seem objectionable and controversial to some.[21,22] However, the reality is that most clients entering treatment for addiction have attempted several times to stop on their own, thereby meeting the second of nine criteria for dependence on a psychoactive substance in the 1987 *Diagnostic and Statistical Manual of Mental Disorders* (3rd ed., revised) (DSM-III-R). To understand how people have tried to terminate drug use on their own before seeking formal treatment, but have failed several times at the attempt, the biological domain must be considered. Particularly when it comes to cocaine (our most addictive drug) and crack (the most addictive form of cocaine), the biological domain explains how compulsive cocaine/crack use patterns develop and lead to repeated failure in terminating crack use. Use of the term *relapse* may capture the cyclical pattern of trying to stop cocaine/crack use—whether for 3 d, 3 wk, or 3 mo—and returning to a compulsive use pattern after failure in accomplishing this goal.

Although we can debate the utility of the term *relapse*, suggest replacing it with concepts like "breaking of a resolution," argue for elimination of the term *relapse*,[21] or define relapse in terms of there having to be a stable period of abstinence of some length before a return to drug use,[22] we may depart from a reality captured in hundreds of case histories and the DSM-III-R criteria for dependence. Much more important than such debate over the use and definition of the term *relapse* is the aim of professionals understanding how the biological domain explains compulsive cocaine/crack use and a cycle of failed attempts to terminate on one's own. Meanwhile, treatment professionals and researchers consider the provision of pharmacological adjuncts and neuronutrients to addicts—in order to ease their experience of intense cravings and withdrawal—as constituting a form of relapse prevention.[20,23]

A proper understanding of this early phenomenon of relapse in response to intense brain-driven cravings for more and more cocaine/crack facilitates empathic response to the addict by the treatment professional. The cocaine/crack dependent client can only receive our empathic delivery of clinical interventions if the treatment professional possesses sound understanding of the following:

1. Chronic use of cocaine/crack leads to neurochemical disruptions in brain functioning;[23,25]
2. Cocaine/crack-induced neurochemical disruptions in brain functioning lead to intense brain-driven cravings; and,[23,25]
3. Intense brain-driven cravings as the key feature of a withdrawal syndrome lock clients into a cycle of self-administration of cocaine/crack and failed attempts to terminate use on their own—whether or not we agree on the use of the term *relapse* to capture early failed attempts to terminate use because of a biological imperative.

An implication of the biological domain is the necessity of delivering neuronutrients or pharmacological adjuncts that serve to restore neurochemical brain functioning and reduce and eliminate intense brain-driven cravings.[20,23–25] In this way, the provision of agents such as bromocriptine, desipramine, and Tropamine™ represent diverse strategies to restore neurochemical brain functioning, reduce intense cravings, induce a state of abstinence, reduce the chances of relapse, reduce departures against medical advice from inpatient programs, and reduce chances of relapse among outpatients.[20,23–25] The successful recovery of the severely dependent cocaine and crack client rests on the provision of one or another of these biological agents. In this way, the biological domain, within a biopsychosocial model of cocaine/crack addiction, is absolutely critical to our achieving empathy with the addict and adequately understanding thc path they have traveled in hitting rock bottom and eventually entering treatment.

The Psychological Domain and Relapse Prevention

Yet our view of cocaine and crack dependence remains incomplete if we do not go beyond the biological domain in our search for possible determinants of relapse or obstacles to successful recovery. Attention to the psychological domain permits our assessment to focus on childhood developmental history, family history, psychiatric history, and observation of defensive and psychological functioning, which may or may not result in additional axis I and axis II diagnoses—via the DSM-III-R—beyond cocaine/crack dependence. Determinants of relapse or obstacles to a successsful recovery may involve a number of factors only understood via elaborate consideration of the psychological domain:

1. Adult child of an alcoholic or dysfunctional family status that seems to carry a higher risk of relapse [26,27];
2. Histories of sexual abuse or molestation that range from 20–70% in the chemically dependent population, or other traumatic abuse, which lead to relapse when newly abstinent clients experience the return of memories, flashbacks, and even the emergence of full-blown posttraumatic stress disorder (PTSD)[28,29];
3. Problems in the regulation of one's affects, self-esteem, impulses, and interpersonal behavior that are rooted in dysfunctional family histories, left clients vulnerable to experience chemicals as extra-reinforcing, and contribute a higher risk of relapse[17,30];
4. Significant psychological trauma experienced as a consequence of crack addiction involving loss of infant custody, loss of jobs, domestic violence, rapes while in crack areas or by "Johns" while prostituting, and witnessing shootings or other drug distribution violence.

Unless clients receive treatment that remediates underlying psychopathology rooted in trauma and childhood development in dysfunctional families, or addresses a PTSD that might emerge when a client is 1 or 9 mo abstinent, the risk of relapse remains high.[17,28] The surprisingly high rates of PTSD in an outpatient crack population supports the need to provide professional psychotherapy.[29]

Professional therapy needs to remediate underlying psychopathology and reduce chances of relapse and symptom substitution. Symptom substitution involves the performance of other compulsive and destructive behaviors—compulsive sex, overeating, gambling, workaholism, shopaholism, etc. The development and implementation of cost-effective models of group therapy remains critical to the successful recovery of a large number of cocaine/crack dependent clients.[31,32]

Only through careful consideration of this psychological domain and the conducting of thorough individualized assessments that pick up relevant psychopathology can clients be matched to professional psychotherapy that reduces chances of relapse by remediating this underlying psychopathology. Just as an implication of considering the biological domain was the need to provide pharmacological adjuncts as treatment that reduces the risk of relapse, an implication of considering the psychological domain is the need to provide professional therapy as treatment that reduces the risk of relapse.

The Social–Environmental Domain and Relapse Prevention

Social learning in a specific environmental context has involved processes of classical and operant conditioning that need to be understood in order to structure treatment programs and interventions that prevent relapse. In the process of classical conditioning, classically conditioned stimuli are the product of numerous cocaine/crack use sessions in which pairing of the drug's pharmacological actions and numerous other stimuli (a crack pipe, a song, a cocaine-using associate, a room, payday, etc.) has occurred. As a result, classically conditioned stimuli (visual sight of a crack pipe, hearing a song, payday) produce the conditioned response of anticipation of the cocaine euphoria, readiness to experience euphoria, craving for cocaine/crack, and relapse. Professionals and clients both need education on this process, and treatment must come to include an evaluation of idiosyncratic determinants of relapse, or idiosyncratic conditioned stimuli that may evoke the conditioned response of cocaine/crack use. (*See* ref. 17 for a detailed discussion.) Adequate treatment will teach clients how to execute alternative behavioral responses, instead of performing a deeply engrained classically conditioned responses, so that a slip or relapse does not occur. Some professionals go as far as to provide extinction trials during inpatient treatment, although treatment outcomes have been dissappointing[33,34] because of persisting idiosyncratic conditioned stimuli to be encountered postinpatient treatment in the real world.

Other professionals recommend a less literal response to the role of conditioned stimuli that can trigger a conditioned response and recommend psychoeducation on determinants of relapse.[17] Psychoeducation permits discussion of alternative behavioral responses to avoid relapse (Wallace, 1991). Clients must learn to anticipate the moment of encountering conditioned stimuli, be prepared at that moment to execute an alternative behavioral response, and understand that each encounter constitutes an extinction trial if chemicals are not used at that moment.

Operant conditioning assists us in understanding from the perspective of the social–environmental domain just how reinforcing the cocaine/crack euphoria has been in establishing a compulsive drug use pattern. The positive reinforcement from the cocaine/crack high has emerged as the most powerful form of reinforcement available from chemicals, when the reinforcing value of cocaine is compared to that of heroin and alcohol in animal laboratory studies.[19] If relapse is to be effectively avoided, clients who are prone to recollection of the positive reinforcement value of the cocaine/crack euphoria need to have alternative sources of positive reinforcement in their lives.

Clinical observation suggests that many clients with alternative sources of positive reinforcement in their lives (a good job, a valued spouse, a car) experience these other sources of positive reinforcement as external controls that place limits on cocaine/crack use.[35] The feared loss of these rewards motivates many clients to seek treatment before hitting even lower levels of rock bottom. Whether clients did hit painfully low levels of rock bottom and lost valued nondrug-related sources of positive reinforcement, or never had many forms of positive reinforcement in their lives, treatment programs are incomplete if they fail to systematically structure sources of positive reinforcement into clients' lives. Relapse prevention can therefore be conceived as including the provision of, or referral for provision of, general equivalency degrees, vocational training, job placement, independent housing, and training in those skills necessary to be able to handle the inevitable stressors associated with employment and intimate relationships.

Negative reinforcement explains how negative-feeling states such as anger or a state of withdrawal can be responded to with administration of cocaine/crack, which ameliorates an aversive state. This results in even more deeply engrained[17] conditioning or learning. An understanding of negative reinforcement can be important in educating professionals and clients on how painful affective states—which were responded to with chemical use—now constitute a challenge when clients have been conditioned to use chemicals to alleviate aversive or painful emotional states. Whether at work or negotiating an intimate relationship, feelings of anger and other painful affects, which inevitably arise in such contexts, need to be responded to without a conditoned response of self-administration of cocaine/crack.

This consideration of the social–environmental domain and how processes of conditioning or learning occur in a specific context carries several implications regarding treatment. Treatment programs may need to guide clients in avoiding classically conditioned responses, as well as responses conditioned through positive and negative reinforcement; we also see the need to structure into clients' lives other sources of positive reinforcement.

In sum, a biopsychosocial approach to cocaine/crack dependence has further assisted in the evolution of our understanding of relapse and ability to prevent relapse episodes effectively. A biopsychosocial approach suggests the necessity of considering biological, psychological, and social domains that play a role in the etiology, maintenance, and treatment of addiction. Relapse prevention must therefore by multidimensional in addressing the biological, psychological, and social domains. An understanding of each of these domains leads to certain implications, involving the need to provide a specific treatment intervention designed to reduce the risk of relapse associated with either a biological, psychological, or social–environmental factor.

A Review of Relevant Research Findings

Beyond the seminal work of Marlatt and Gordon,[3] the views of frontline treatment professionals who have observed and described the process of relapse, and the utility of a biopsychosocial approach with its varied implications, our contemporary understanding of relapse has also evolved in light of important research findings. However, a limited amount of research shedding light on the process and determinants of relapse in cocaine/crack dependent clients appears to date in the literature.

Outcome Evaluation Research and the Prevention of Relapse

Among the limited outcome evaluation research that has been conducted specifically with cocaine- and crack-using populations, the work of Washton[22] indicates the critical role of relapse prevention in producing relatively successful treatment outomes for this difficult population. Washton's research includes a small sample (n = 60) and has methodological limitations. This data suggests that "employed cocaine and crack addicts can be treated successfully in inpatient or outpatient programs that are followed by intensive aftercare treatment emphasizing relapse prevention" (p. 147). Follow-up of 60 consecutive admissions to the Washton Institute indicated that 40 entered directly without prior inpatient treatment, and 20 entered outpatient treatment after completing an inpatient program. Washton found that "68% of the outpatients and 64% of the inpatients were abstinent at 6- to 24-mo follow-up according to urine tests and clinical interviews" (p.147). Even among what are considered successful outcomes, a slip to their drug of choice (33%) or to some other chemical use (23%) characterized their recovery. Suggestive of the more difficult treatment challenge associated with smoking of cocaine alkaloid (free-base or crack), lower abstinence follow-up rates (58%) characterized the cocaine smokers when compared to the better follow-up abstinence rates found with cocaine snorters (78%).

Washton's data is important in clarifying how the majority of cocaine and crack dependent clients will experience a slip or return to some chemical use. Moreover, when clients are involved in a comprehensive and intensive treatment regime, which includes urine testing, relapse prevention education, and therapeutic support, a slip does not have to result in a full-blown relapse.

Although there is other suggestive research,[36] in general, methodological problems limit the usefulness of this data.[17] What does emerge from the research done to date is that cocaine and crack clients require a continuum of care spanning the initial 6 mo of recovery, which provides intensive and comprehensive services—whether the care includes inpatient followed by outpatient, inpatient detoxificaton followed by a residential TC stay for the severely dependent, or outpatient treatment alone.[17] The provision of relapse prevention is the most critical treatment component, and even with its provision, a slip or relapse must be anticipated, picked up via routine or random urine testing, and openly discussed and analyzed within both group and individual therapy settings to avoid its reoccurrence.

Evidence of a Critical Period for Providing Relapse Prevention

The importance of providing intensive and comprehensive treatment services spanning the initial 6 mo of recovery, finds further support from the research of Wallace.[15,17] Although data was not obtained within a formal outcome evaluation study, of the 288 clients treated on an inpatient detoxifaction unit over a 2-yr period, a total of 35 clients returned for a second detoxification following relapse. Following Marlatt's[3] use of the microanalysis of the relapse episode via questionnaire, Wallace[15] used a clinical relapse interview to identify the determinants of clients' relapse episodes.

An analysis of time to relapse[16,17] showed that after a 14-d hospital stay 31.4% of clients relapse within a week, 24.3% relapse between 2 wk and 1 mo, 20% relapse between 60 and 90 d, 8.6% relapse between 3.5 and 4.5 mo, and 5.7% relapse between 6 and 7 mo; totaling 94.3% experiencing a relapse before 6 mo expire since completion of inpatient detoxification. Within the first 90 d post-detox, 76% relapse. This data is unique insofar as the sample was primarily composed of severely dependent crack cocaine smokers. The findings are significant in pinpointing the initial 90 d of recovery, as well as the initial 6 mo, as a critical period in which interventions need to be delivered to assist clients in avoiding a slip or relapse.

Psychological and Environmental Determinants of Relapse

Other data arising from Wallace's[15,17] microanalysis of relapse episodes (n = 35) indicate that the determinants of relapse fall into a psychological/personality domain covering internal factors, as well as an environmental/interpersonal domain covering external factors—creating a total of 11 categories. Determinants of relapse involving internal factors include painful emotional states (40%), denial (and denial exacerbated by narcissistic inflation) (28.5%), failure to enter arranged aftercare treatment (37.14%), refusal of aftercare treatment (11.42%), and drug craving (5.7%). External determinants of relapse, which psychologically vulnerable patients handle poorly, include: encounters with environmental stimuli of people, places, and things (34.28%); interpersonal stress (24.38%); escalation to drug of choice after use of chemicals (14.28%); failing the hard test of handling money, where money is a classically conditioned stimulus (11.42%); homelessness or lack of family support (14.28%); and, service delivery system shortcomings reflected in long waiting lists to enter a residential TC and policies whereby TCs refuse to admit individuals with psychiatric or medical problems. Thus, these findings support a model that views a relapse episode as the product of psychological vulnerability interacting with encounters with external environmental stimuli.

Evidence of Multiple Determinants of Relapse

Perhaps most importantly, relapse involves multideterminants that subtly interact. The vast majority of clients (85.7%) experienced relapse episodes involving multideterminants, with most experiencing a combination of two (37.13%) or three (40%) determinants. The majority of relapse episodes involve both psychological and environmental determinants. Most common combinations of determinants include painful emotional states from the psychological domain and interpersonal stress from the environmental domain (20%). Also commonly occurring in tandem is either failure to enter, or refusal of, aftercare treatment together with narcissistic denial (22.8%).[15,17]

These findings give rise to a model of relapse prevention. Other models of relapse prevention, such as that producing the follow-up results of Washton discussed earlier, merit review in the next section as well.

Models of Relapse Prevention

Models of relapse prevention have been designed specifically to meet the needs of the new and challenging cocaine and crack population of the 1980s[14,15,17,22,25,37] whereas other models were designed for alcoholics or other addicts, but often find extension to the chemically dependent in general.[28,38–41] This section focuses primarily on models of relapse prevention specifically designed or modified for use with the cocaine and crack dependent, providing a review of the work of Wallace,[15,17] Washton,[14,22] Rawson,[37,42] and Gorski.[38,43]

Wallace's Model of Relapse Prevention

Among the models of relapse prevention described in the literature, Wallace's[15,17] model was designed specifically in light of her research findings on the determinants of relapse summarized earlier. Wallace strove within the context of twice weekly 1-h groups held on the inpatient detoxification unit at Interfaith Medical Center, Brooklyn, New York, to deliver psychoeducation designed to prevent relapse when severely dependent crack smokers left 14-d inpatient treatment. A total of 29 interventions educate clients regarding the 11 categories of determinants of relapse falling under psychological and environmental domains. Psychoeducation also covers the nature of the first 90 d and 6 mo of abstinence as a critical period in which involvement in adequate aftercare treatment and the use of alternative behavioral strategies need to be adhered to in order to avoid relapse. Within this model of relapse, clinicians must be active educators who utilize a multifaceted clinical technique combining the cognitive–behavioral, psychodynamic, and metaphorical forms of communication as crucial elements. Detailed description of what exactly clinicians should do and say within the context of a psychoeducational group delivering this model of relapse prevention appears elsewhere.[15,17]

The strength of this model of relapse prevention involves the extent to which it is derived from findings on the determinants of relapse for a sample of compulsive crack cocaine smokers. The model also maximizes the power of graphic and visual metaphors in bypassing defenses, resistance, and any subtle cognitive deficits clients may possess from chronic chemical use. The model maximizes even a brief 14-d inpatient period as an opportunity to impact patients' consciousness and educate them to determinants of relapse to which patients just like them succumbed. The model can be adapted to other settings (outpatient, residential TC), the interventions delivered in other modalitites (individual therapy), and with other populations (adult children of alcoholic and other dysfunctional families). A weakness of the model is that it does not provide for sufficient time for rehearsal of alternative behavioral strategies, and no outcome evaluation research to date has assessed its efficacy in preventing relapse.

Wallace[44] also cautioned that implementation of this psychoeducational model of relapse prevention remains incomplete if a treatment program does not provide neuronutrients or pharmacological adjuncts to address intense cravings and a withdrawal syndrome. Also, consistent with the approach to relapse Young[28] endorsed, a significant subset of clients need more than psychoeducation on the impact of childhood sexual abuse, physical abuse, or other trauma. Such clients require professional therapy in group or individual treatment modalities, which will remediate underlying psychopathology stemming from their trauma. Ultimately relapse prevention must be conceived of as including long-term involvement in professional therapy, which remediates underlying psychopathology, going well beyond the 6-mo critical period of initial abstinence in which intensive and comprehensive treatment[14,17,42] should be delivered to all addicts—with or without trauma.

Washton's Model of Relapse Prevention

Among the models providing adequately intensive and comprehensive cocaine and crack treatment, the outpatient model offered at the Washton Institute in New York City stands out as state-of-the-art. The various elements of the treatment program have been discussed in detail elsewhere.[14,17,22] Briefly, the program includes provision of relapse prevention, urine testing, individual sessions, psychoeducation for clients and family members, group therapy, 12-step group involvement, and family/couples counseling.

As a comprehensive program offering numerous services, this model within itself offers numerous safeguards against relapse. As Washton and Stone-Washton[22] explained, a highly structured outpatient regimen replaces habitual drug use with habitual attendance at the program (p. 139). Also key to preventing relapse is first establishing abstinence via short-term goals, frequent supportive contact, urine testing, external controls (no access to bank accounts), and use of other support systems such as 12-step groups. Clients also learn how to avoid cocaine triggers, which include people, places, things, and emotional states. Techniques are also taught regarding how to manage cravings.

Contrary to the view of professionals who believe that with cocaine and crack clients in particular relapse prevention needs to begin on d 1 of treatment,[17,45] Washton and Stone-Washton believed that "only when abstinence is firmly established can the focus of treatment shift to relapse prevention" (p. 143). Consistent with diverse professional views on how to define relapse,[21] Washton and Stone-Washton[22] believed that unless a client has at least 3 mo of solid abstinence a return to drug use should be viewed as continuation of a drug use pattern and not relapse (p. 143). In fact, these authors felt that "giving vulnerable, marginally motivated cocaine addicts long lists of relapse warning signs is tantamount to giving them a menu of excuses to get high" (p. 144).

Obviously Wallace's[15,17] delivery of relapse prevention in psychoeducational groups (described earlier), which in effect presents to clients a list of 11 common determinants of relapse to which 35 clients just like themselves succumbed, flies in the face of Washton and Stone-Washton's caution. Yet, as we saw, Wallace[15,17] strove to recommend and teach alternative behavioral strategies that clients must execute to avoid a relapse for each of the 11 categories of determinants of relapse. Also, Todd[45] in describing an outcome evaluation study, which was transformed into a study reporting the characteristics of clients who drop out of treatment, emphasized that relapse prevention should have started on d 1 of treatment. Clearly, only clinicians' experiences, the data of their observations, the modifications they make for specific populations in specific settings, and changes made in service delivery for individual clients with specific characteristics determines what they end up recommending. Only formal outcome evaluation studies comparing various models of relapse prevention can reveal which models of relapse prevention are most efficacious for different kinds of cocaine and crack addicts.

Nonetheless, Washton's model of relapse prevention, which has helped to produce fairly good treatment outcomes, involves the following elements in an outpatient setting treating employed and motivated cocaine and crack clients: explanation of the terms *jump* (a deliberate and preplanned use of drugs), *slip* (which is accidental), and *relapse* (return to pretreatment level of drug use). The model also involves dealing therapeutically with patients who experience a slip, following Marlatt in treating slips as an opportunity to learn. Also, assessment of cocaine-related changes in sexuality occur to avoid a relapse involving the closely linked cocaine addiction and compulsive sexuality frequently found in combination in their population (70%).

As mentioned in the earlier section of this chapter on research findings, the Washton Institute's program has suggestive research regarding the efficacy and success of their treatment approach (68% abstinent with outpatient treatment alone at 6- to 24-mo follow-up). We can only wonder if their greater success with cocaine snorters (78%) vs cocaine alkaloid smokers (free-base or crack) (58%) indicates that the smokers needed earlier and more extensive relapse prevention such as the multidimensional approach to relapse prevention designed and recommended for crack smokers.[44] Or, a careful analysis of Washton's overall treatment model suggests that a codified and elaborate psychoeducational curriculum to which every client is exposed via workbooks and films constitutes an essential form of relapse prevention, which is delivered to clients early in the treatment process. Washton's psychoeducation covers in elaborate fashion a variety of cocaine triggers, how conditioning establishes such triggers, what strategies do not work in coping with cravings, and numerous strategies for successfully coping with cocaine cravings. A strong argument can be made that this high caliber and comprehensive psychoeducational curriculum does indeed constitute extensive relapse prevention, despite Washton and Stone-Washton's[22] assertion that relapse prevention only begins much later in treatment after several months when abstinence has been firmly established.

Clearly the field of chemical dependency must continue to evolve and address current controversies in the field such as the lack of consensus on when to use the term *relapse*, as well as tendencies to recommend the same treatment for everyone. Only carefully designed and methodologically rigorous outcome evaluation research can determine the characteristics of programs and of individual cocaine and crack clients that when matched together produce the best treatment outcomes. Until such research is done, Washton's model of relapse prevention emerges as a key component of a generally successful state-of-the-art treatment model. A refreshing strength of this model is the emphasis on jumps, which is important in educating clients regarding possible outright decisions to get high, and the recommendation to assess drug-related changes in sexuality in search for a compulsive sexuality.

Rawson's Model of Relapse Prevention

Although attributed to Rawson, the Matrix Center in California developed an outpatient model in 1983 for cocaine abusers that reflected the collective knowledge and expertise of leading addictions specialists across the nation.[37,42] The resulting neurobehavioral treatment for cocaine dependency stands as yet another state-of-the-art treatment model that provides comprehensive and intensive services. Services provided include individual sessions, group therapy, family therapy, 12-step group involvement, urine testing, and relapse prevention. The delivery of interventions follows a timetable of recovery, or stages of recovery in which clients' experiences in emotional, cognitive, behavioral, and relationship realms are addressed in highly structured individual therapy sessions with a professional therapist. Treatment is intensive in so far as clients come to treatment 4–5 d per wk over the first 6 mo of recovery, and also attend a weekly group from mo 7–12. As with the Washton Institute model, the provision of such highly structured, comprehensive, and intensive services during the 6-mo critical period identified by Wallace's[15,17] research serves to reduce chances of relapse.

The model of relapse prevention provided within Rawson's Matrix Center program has benefited from the prior work of numerous professionals and involves the relapse prevention group and the relapse analysis process. The relapse prevention group is attended from mo 2–6, while the weekly group from mo 7–12 also addresses relapse issues. The highly structured long-term group provides information about relapse and relapse prevention, while covering specific topics—sexual readjustment, serenity prayer, relapse prevention, monthly review, cocaine dreams, reestablishing trust, keeping a distance from relapse, relapse justification, balance, truthfulness, motivation, fatigue, responsibility for recovery, addictive behavior, island building, guilt and shame, disinhibiting drugs, and holidays.

Therapists have been trained in how to handle a relapse if it occurs via a structured exercise codified in a worksheet, occurring in individual sessions immediately after the relapse. The worksheet includes categories in which relevant events may have led to relapse: career events, personal events, treatment events, drug/alcohol related behaviors, behavioral patterns, relapse cognitions, and health habits status. This exercise identifies events leading up to the relapse so that clues for prevention of future relapse can be identified, however relapse does not mean failure. Family sessions may also be held to recant an analysis of the relapse episode. Clients are taught to recognize relapse as a process so that they can stop or interrupt the process before active chemical use occurs. After a relapse, extra precautions are taken for vulnerable clients, extending for several weeks. The definition of relapse that Rawson and his colleagues follow is that "relapses are defined as episodes of cocaine use that occur after periods of extended sobriety (usually a month or more). If the episodes of drug use are close together, the client needs to focus on stopping drug use as opposed to avoiding relapses"[37] (p. 167). Clearly, diverse professional views on how to define relapse prevail.

A major strength of this model of relapse prevention, as well as the overall Matrix Center treatment program, is that structured manuals for training therapists permits consistent delivery of services, which is ideal for research and replicating the model[37]; outcome evaluation research is currently underway. We must wonder to what extent this model recognizes that different clients need different kinds of interventions that may go beyond a consistent package delivered in a structured fashion by therapists—such as the provision of professional therapy to address childhood trauma (sexual abuse, physical abuse) or adult trauma in the crack culture from battering and rapes.

For employed clients with good insurance or the ability to pay on average the $4500[17] cost of treatment, psychosocial functioning may be such that individualized assessments do not uncover significant trauma requiring an individualized plan of professional therapy. On the other hand, Rawson's experiences with "hard-core" crack users who have been on a binge in the streets for a long time has convinced him of the need to place them in the hospital for 3–5 d prior to entrance into the treatment program. At one Matrix facility there is even a sliding scale with a monthly cost of $25 for those at the bottom of the scale.[42]

Rawson[42] stated that many "of these cocaine abusers won't be able to get off the drug no matter what treatment they receive. These hard-core abusers may be mentally ill, are often heavily involved in criminal activities, and generally suffer severe societal problems such as chronic unemployment" (p. 10). However, if we consider the wisdom of Marlatt,[46] upon failure in even the best outpatient treatment program, clinical assessment turns toward consideration of placing patients in even more intensive inpatient and long-term residential programs.

Since the overall psychosocial functioning of clients varies as does their characteristics and demographics, despite an impressive program and relapse prevention model, Rawson's approach may require additional components for some clients. Following Wallace,[17] for compulsive crack cocaine smokers, treatment needs to address the biological, psychological, and social–environmental domains, respectively, via provision of pharmacological adjuncts or neuronutrients to address craving/withdrawal, psychoeducation and professional therapy to address psychopathology, and delivery of services to build skills so clients can experience economic and interpersonal relationship rewards. Thus, a weakness of any relapse prevention model may lie in its failure to address all of the domains within a biopsychosocial approach. Even outpatient programs may find that the provision of neuronutrients such as Tropamine™ can reduce relapse rates[25] when the biological domain is addressed.

Future research has to determine whether the provision of professional therapy in cost-effective group, or individual therapy contexts, which does address clients' psychopathology and trauma, reduces the risk of relapse as some suggest[17,28,47]; these approaches attempt to address adequately the psychological domain. Meanwhile, residential therapeutic communities long ago recognized the critical role of addressing the social–environmental domain through incorporation of vocational training, job placement, and independent housing into the therapeutic process in order to facilitate the recovery of their severely dependent and debilitated clients. Again, only research that examines the characteristics of individual clients and program models, which when matched together produce the best treatment outcomes, can clarify for which clients certain combinations of treatment are most efficacious in reducing the risk of relapse.

Gorski's Model of Relapse Prevention

Gorski[38] has developed a model of relapse prevention that was initially developed through his work with primarily alcoholics. Through his CENAPS corporation, Gorski has developed a relapse prevention certification program that attempts to draw a national body of treatment professionals and prepare them to initiate a relapse prevention program in their treatment setting when they return from his training. Thus, his wisdom gained through years of work with primarily an alcoholic population finds extension to the more recent cocaine and crack population, while chemical dependency treatment units across the nation may implement his model as professional workers receive the CENAPS relapse prevention ceritication.

One concept arising from the CENAPS model is the notion of structuring a primary recovery program. The primary recovery program teaches

1. That chemical dependency is a biopsychosocial disease;

2. The concept of lifelong abstinence;
3. The importance of developing an ongoing recovery program; and
4. Covers the diagnosis and treatment of other problems or conditions.

For clients in primary recovery, it is not appropriate to speak of the use of alcohol or drugs in terms of relapse, but of a continuation of an untreated disease progression.[38] Furthermore, Gorski[38] felt that clients who have not yet accomplished the four goals of the primary recovery program need to be separated from those clients who already understand their disease but are unable to maintain abstinence. Thus, in the CENAPS model, clients are separated into two groups and treated separately based on whether they are new to treatment or have experienced a relapse. For appropriate candidates who already accomplished the four goals of primary recovery, but have relapsed, the process of relapse prevention therapy is initiated.

Education on warning signs and the related process of relapse and recovery covers six levels:

1. Abstaining from alcohol and other drugs;
2. Establishing a recovery centered social life so that one separates from people, places, and things that promote chemical use;
3. Stopping compulsive behavior that suppress awareness of painful feelings and irrational thoughts;
4. Learning how to manage feelings without resorting to compulsive behaviors or use of chemicals;
5. Learning to change addictive-thinking patterns that create painful feelings and self-defeating behaviors; and
6. Identifying and changing mistaken beliefs, or core beliefs, about self, others, and the world that promote irrational thinking (p. 128).[28]

In addition, Gorski[28] identified the following nine principles that form the basis of specific relapse prevention therapy procedures.

1. The principle of self-regulation states that the risk of relapse will decrease as the capacity to self-regulate their thinking, feeling, memory, judgment, and behavior increases; this guides attempts to stabilize the client through detoxification or provision of a drug-free environment, as therapists challenge irrational thinking and plan for what to do if a return to chemical use occurs (pp. 128,129).
2. The principle of integration states that risk of relapse will decrease as the level of conscious understanding and acceptance of situations and events that led to past relapses increases; this leads to a careful self-

assessment of chemical use and one's relapse history (p. 129).

3. The principle of understanding states that the risk of relapse will decrease as the understanding of the general factors that cause relapse increases; this guides therapeutic efforts to provide education on relapse (p. 130).
4. The principle of self-knowledge states that risk of relapse will decrease as the patients ability to recognize personal relapse warning signs increases; clients identify personal behaviors, beliefs, and triggers that are warning signs of possible relapse.
5. The principle of coping skills states that risk of relapse decreases as ability to manage relapse warning signs increases; clients learn to manage their personal warning signs by, for example, rehearsing coping strategies in face of high-risk situations.
6. The principle of change states that risk of relapse will decrease as the relationship between relapse warning signs and recovery program recommendations increases; clients engage in recovery planning where they develop a schedule of activities that help them recognize and manage warning signs as they develop in sobriety (p. 132).
7. The principle of awareness states that risk of relapse decreases as use of daily inventory techniques designed to identify relapse warning signs increases; clients learn to monitor daily their compliance with their recovery program, checking for the emergence of warning signs (p. 132).
8. The principle of significant others states that risk of relapse decreases as the responsible involvement of significant others in recovery from codependency and in the relapse prevention planning process increases; family and others must get involved in relapse prevention planning (p. 132).
9. The principle of maintenance states that the risk of relapse decreases if the relapse prevention plan is regularly updated during the first 3 yr of sobriety; updating moves from monthly, to quarterly, to semiannually, to annually with time over 3 yr, as clients revise warning signs and management strategies (pp. 132,133).

Gorski[28] asserted that this model not only guides therapeutic interventions, but can also guide research evaluations. A strength of the model is its comprehensiveness, provision of a continuum of care and relapse prevention strategies over the course of the first to third year of recovery, and attention to improving clients' self-regulation and coping strategies. This model also attends to the need to avoid symptom substitution or the emergence of other compulsive and destructive behaviors. Although originally designed for recidivist alcoholics, this model is being extended to cocaine/crack dependent clients, whereas Gorski (1991) also educated professionals and clients on cocaine craving and relapse as he also embraced in general a biopsychosocial understanding of chemical disease.

Conclusion

This chapter has emphasized the critical importance of relapse prevention in the treatment of the cocaine and crack dependent. The cocaine and crack epidemic of the 1980s challenged professionals to utilize their observations in building further on the important work of Marlatt and Gordon,[3] which established the task of preventing relapse as central to the treatment of varied addictions. Professionals responded to the cocaine/crack treatment challenge by refining a multifaceted clinical technique that combines psychoeducation, cognitive–behavioral, psychodynamic, and metaphorical elements. Meanwhile, biopsychosocial models remind us of the need to forge an integrated theoretical paradigm to guide the provision of treatments. The scant research available sheds further light on the relapse process, determinants of relapse, and frequency of the occurrence of relapse that permits the refinement of relapse prevention models. Relapse prevention models designed in light of the characteristics of the cocaine/crack dependent clients being serviced within various programs have been reviewed. An examination of models of relapse prevention indicates that professionals differ on their definitions of relapse, sense of when to invoke the term *relapse,* decisions regarding to whom one delivers relapse prevention, conceptions of what constitutes relapse prevention, and when this relapse prevention education should be delivered.

This author follows researchers who emphasize the biological basis of addiction[20,23] and deploy the term *relapse* to refer to an early and immediate return to cocaine/crack use after just a brief attempt at abstinence during an inpatient hospital stay. On the other hand, Washton,[14,22] Rawson,[37] and Gorski[38] are more conservative in their use of the term *relapse,* reserving use of the term for those individuals who have clearly experienced some period of abstinence ranging from one to several months. Prior to this several-month period expiring, use of chemicals is seen as continuation of a drug use pattern.

Because of this view, Washton, Rawson, and Gorski all delayed the provision of relapse prevention for some period of time, although this period varies. And, because of the basic view of relapse captured in a definition of relapse, which distinguishes between continuation of a drug use pattern vs a relapse after primary recovery goals were pursued, Gorski in fact separated those who are new to treatment from those who have already been through treatment, experience a relapse, but already worked on the primary tasks of recovery. However, I have emphasized that the provision of psychoeducation that occurs early in treatment, and is a part of Gorski's primary recovery education, may in a subtle but powerful way convey essential relapse prevention education. Washton also provided vital psychoeducation via workbooks and films, which occurs early in treatment and may nonetheless convey important relapse prevention education. The same can be argued for the approach of Rawson. This suggests lack of agreement as to what constitutes relapse prevention or relapse prevention education. Wallace clearly saw the provision of psychoeducation as a valid vehicle for delivering information that will assist in the avoidance of a slip or relapse.

On the other hand, Wallace also believed that cocaine and crack clients in particular need relapse prevention to begin on d 1 of treatment. On the other hand, Gorski separated out those new to treatment into a primary recovery program that does not systematically follow the nine principles that guide treatment for those who have already experienced treatment as well as a relapse. Clearly, Wallace may have felt a different kind of pressure to prepare a new crack dependent population for what was to follow a 14-d inpatient detoxification program, whereas Gorski had been influenced by his primary work with alcoholics who returned to 28-d inpatient programs after a painful relapse and clearly needed something different the second or fourth time around. Thus, an additional issue involves the extent to which clinicians differ in how they structure their models of relapse prevention in light of being in an inpatient or outpatient setting with clients possessing varying characteristics and chemical use backgrounds.

Gorski and Wallace presented a conception of relapse and share some agreement on the kind of activities that should also be subsumed under relapse prevention. The tasks of improving self-regulation, improving management of painful feelings, and addressing tendencies to engage in other destructive and compulsive behaviors are all seen as falling within relapse prevention activities, even if this means involvement with recovery activities that will address irrational cognitions, or remediate underlying poor self-regulatory capacities, or treat underlying psychopathology. Washton and Rawson deemphasized the need to remediate underlying psychopathology to reduce chances of relapse, as Gorski and Wallace stressed.

Rawson and Washton shared agreement in structuring intensive and comprehensive outpatient programs that not only emphasize relapse prevention, but are also highly structured programs that deliver specific interventions in light of the phase of recovery a client negotiates. The points of convergence and divergence among professionals create a necessary tension that promotes the articulation of research questions that may alone answer the questions raised.

Future Directions in Research and Relapse Prevention

Important questions raised involve the rationale of using the term *relapse* to describe failed attempts to stop on one's own, and the rationale for using the term *relapse* to capture failed attempts to stop on one's own because of a biologically based craving and withdrawal syndrome. To the extent that provision of pharmacological adjuncts and neuronutrients has permitted the avoidance of relapse and decreased departures against medical advice, many would argue that this point has already been validated in research,[17,19,20,23] even if some clinicians fail to emphasize and recognize the biological basis of cocaine/crack addiction. This author has embraced the importance of following a biopsychosocial model of cocaine and crack addiction with its implications for relapse prevention, as articulated in this chapter. Although disagreement and tension can promote thought and the articulation of research questions, a biopsychosocial model may be most effective in drawing attention to the need for a multidimensional view of relapse prevention that arises from a consideration of biological, psychological, and social–environmental domains.

Disparate rationales regarding when to deliver relapse prevention and to whom we should deliver these interventions can either receive confirmation or rejection through carefully designed outcome evaluation research. A basic question to be explored is the following: What are the characteristics of individual clients and of individual programs that when matched together produce the best long-term treatment outcomes? Follow-up periods may need to extend beyond the traditional 6- and even 18-mo recovery period, while careful attention must be paid to the definition of a slip, relapse, and the emergence of some substituting symptoms. A clear statement of a definition of a slip or relapse—if not agreement on a definition—remains critical in research studies if a future metaanalysis of relapse studies is to answer this question adequately.

Future research also needs to determine the most cost-effective relapse prevention models and strategies for matching clients to specific relapse prevention models or treatments that best meet their needs and characteristics. The field of chemical dependency must move beyond recommending the same treatments for everyone. And, even though Gorski gave a different treatment to individuals in light of a past attempt at recovery, more sophisticated client-to-treatment matching strategies are needed based on the chemical on which one is dependent and numerous other client characteristics. The distinctiveness of aspects of addiction to cocaine vs crack, or crack vs alcohol, or methamphetamine vs crack, must be understood as this influences the course of addiction and recovery. This may be important even as we decide to treat diverse addicts on one unit, or in one setting, and talk about chemical dependency in general.

The highly structured treatments of Washton and Rawson similarly must explore through research to what extent clients within programs may or may not need all of the comprehensive and intensive services they provide, or which clients need yet something more. As we saw, Washton and Rawson deemphasized the need to remediate underlying psychopathology to reduce chances of relapse, whereas Gorski and Wallace stressed this task as being central to avoiding relapse and symptom substitution. Are there clients that attend the Washton or Rawson treatment programs and, while receiving highly structured relapse prevention education and strategies, end up being treatment failures because of insufficient remediation of underlying psychopathology? In this way, future research must clarify the distinct characteristics of clients and of programs that when matched together produce the best treatment outcomes. And only a thorough individualized assessment that identifies multiple, distinct client characteristics can permit this kind of research question being adequately answered. We may certainly find that for even a single global variable, such as psychopathology, attention to level or degree of psychopathology must be maintained in future research, consistent with past ground-breaking research.[48]

The stimulus provided by the 1980s cocaine and crack epidemic has stimulated growth in the field of chemical dependency and relapse prevention so that we now possess a multifaceted clinical technique and integrated theoretical paradigm within a biopsychosocial model. Hopefully, the field can effectively answer pertinent research questions and implement indicated improvements in service delivery.

References

[1]W. A. Hunt, L. W. Barnett, and L. G. Branch (1971) Relapse rates in addiction programs. *J. Clin. Psychol.* **27,** 455–456.

[2]C. Cummings, J. Gordon, and G. A. Marlatt (1980) Relapse: Strategies of prevention and prediction, in *The Addictive Behaviors*. W. R. Miller, ed. Pergamon, Oxford, UK.

[3]G. A. Marlatt and J. R. Gordon (1985) *Relapse Prevention.* Guilford, New York.

[4]B. C. Wallace (1989b) Relapse prevention in psychoeducational groups for compulsive crack cocaine smokers. *J. Subst. Abuse Treatment* **6,** 229–239.

[5]A. L. Anker and T. J. Crowley (1982) Use of contingency contracting in specialty clinics for cocaine abuse, in *Problems of Drug Dependence 1981* (NIDA Research Monograph 41). L. S. Harris, ed. US Government Printing Office. Washington, DC.

[6]M. S. Gold (1984) *800-Cocaine*. Bantam, New York.

[7]N. Stone, M. Fromme, and D. Kagan (1984) *Cocaine: Seduction and Solution*. Potter, New York.

[8]D. E. Smith and D. R. Wesson (1985) Cocaine abuse and treatment: An overview, in *Treating the Cocaine Abuser*. D. E. Smith and D. R. Wesson, eds. Hazeldon Foundation, Center City, MN.

[9]D. R. Wesson and D. E. Smith (1985) Cocaine: Treatment perspectives, in *Cocaine Use in America: Epidemiologic and Clinical Perspectives* (NIDA Research Monograph 61). N. J. Kozel and E. H. Adams, eds. US Government Printing Office, Washington, DC.

[10]H. I. Spitz (1987) Cocaine abuse: Therapeutic group approaches, in *Cocaine Abuse: New Directions in Treatment and Research*. H. I. Spitz and J. J. Rosecan, eds. Brunner/Mazel, New York.

[11]H. I. Spitz and S. T. Spitz (1987) Family therapy of cocaine abuse, in *Cocaine Abuse: New Directions in Treatment and Research*. H. I. Spitz and J. J. Rosecan, eds. Brunner/Mazel, New York.

[12]R. M. Kertzner (1987) Individual Psychotherapy of Cocaine Abuse, in *Cocaine Abuse: New Directions in Treatment and Research*. H. I. Spitz and J. S. Rosecan, eds. Brunner/Mazel, New York.

[13]A. M. Washton (1987) Outpatient treatment techniques, in *Cocaine: A Clinicians Handbook*. A. M. Washton and M. S. Gold, eds. Guilford, New York.

[14]A. M. Washton (1989) *Cocaine Addiction: Treatment, Recovery, and Relapse Prevention*. W. W. Norton, New York.

[15]B. C. Wallace (1989a) Psychological and environmental determinants of relapse in crack cocaine smokers. *J. Subst. Abuse Treatment* **6,** 95–106.

[16]D. M. Donovan and G. A. Marlatt, eds. (1988) *Assessment of Addictive Behaviors.* Guilford, New York.

[17]B. C. Wallace (1991) *Crack cocaine: A practical treatment approach for the chemically dependent.* Brunner/Mazel, New York.

[18]E. J. Chiauzzi (1991) *Preventing Relapse in the Addictions: A Biopsychosocial Approach.* Pergamon, New York.

[19]H. I. Spitz and J. J. Rosecan eds. (1987) *Cocaine Abuse: New Directions in Treatment and Research.* Brunner/Mazel, New York.

[20]P. Herridge and M. Gold (1988) Pharmacological Adjuncts in the Treatment of Opiod and Cocaine Addicts. *J. Psychoactive Drugs* **20,** 233–242.

[21]M. Gossop (1989) *Relapse and Addictive Behavior.* Tavistok, New York.

[22]A. M. Washton and N. Stone-Washton (1990) Abstinence and relapse in outpatient cocaine addicts. *J. Psychoactive Drugs* **22,** 135–147.

[23]M. C. Trachtenberg and K. Blum (1988) Improvement of cocaine-induced neuromodulator deficits by the neuronurtient tropamine. *J. Psychoactive Drugs* **20,** 315–331.

[24]F. Gawin (1989) Treatment of crack and cocaine abusers, paper presented 10/24/89, at the "What Work"s: An International Perspective on Drug Abuse Treatment and Prevention Research Conference, New York.

[25]R. J. Brown, K. Blum, and M. C. Trachtenberg (1990) Neurodynamics of relapse prevention: A neuronutrient approach to outpatient DUI offenders. *J. Psychoactive Drugs* **22,** 173–187.

[26]B. Wanck (1985) Treatment of adult children of alcoholics. *Carrier Found. Lett.* **109,** 6.

[27]B. C. Wallace (1990a) Crack cocaine smokers as adult children of alcoholics: the dysfunctional family link. *J. Subst. Abuse Treatment* **7,** 89–100.

[28]E. B. Young (1990) The role of incest issues in relapse. *J. Psychoactive Drugs* **22,** 249–258.

[29]M. Fullilove (1991) July, Personal Communication.

[30]E. J. Khantzian (1985) On the psychological predisposition for opiate and stimulant dependence. *Psychiatry Lett.,* **3,** 1.

[31]B. C. Wallace (in press) The therapeutic community as a treatment modality and the role of the professional consultant: spotlight on Damon House, in *The Chemically Dependent: Phases of Treatment and Recovery.* B. C. Wallace, ed. Brunner/Mazel, New York.

[32]E. J. Khantzian, K. S. Halliday, and W. E. McAuliffe (1990) *Addiction and the Vulnerable Self: Modified Dynamic Group Therapy for Substance Abusers.* Guilford, New York.

[33]A. Childress, R. Ehrman, A. T. McLellan, and C. O'Brian (1988) Conditioned

craving and arousal in cocaine addiction: A preliminary report, in *Problems of Drug Dependence, 1987* L.S. Harris, ed. U.S. Government Printing Office, Washington, DC.

[34]A. R. Childress, A. T. McLellan, R. Ehrman, and C. P. O'Brien (1988) Classically conditioned responses in opiod and cocaine dependence: A role in relapse? in *Learning Factors in Substance Abuse* (NIDA Research Monograph 84). B. A. Ray, ed., US Government Printing Office, Washington, DC.

[35]B. C. Wallace (1990b) Crack addiction: Treatment and recovery issues. *Contemporary Drug Problems* (Spring) 1990.

[36]R. A. Rawson, J. L. Obert, M. J. McCann, and A. J. Mann (1986) *Cocaine Treatment Outcome: Cocaine Use Following Inpatient, Outpatient, and No Treatment* (NIDA Research Monograph 67). National Institute on Drug Abuse, Rockville, MD.

[37]R. A. Rawson, J. L. Obert, M. J. McCann, M. S. Smith, and W. Ling (1990) Neurobehavioral treatment for cocaine dependency. *J. Psychoactive Drugs* **22,** 159–171.

[38]T. T. Gorski (1990) The Cenaps model of relapse prevention: Basic principles and procedures. *J. Psychoactive Drugs* **22,** 125–133.

[39]H. M. Annis (1990) Relapse to substance abuse: Empirical findings within a cognitive-social learning approach *J. Psychoactive Drugs* **22,** 117–124.

[40]M. E. Larimer and G. A. Marlatt (1990) Application of relapse prevention with moderation goals *J. Psychoactive Drugs* **22,** 189–195.

[41]H. D. Weiner, M. C. Wallen, and G. L. Zankowski (1990) Culture and social class as intervening variables in relapse prevention with chemically dependent women. *J. Psychoactive Drugs* **22,** 239–248.

[42]R. Rawson (1990) Cut the crack: the policymaker's guide to cocaine treatment. *Policy Rev.* (Winter) 10–19.

[43]T. Gorski (1991) Cocaine, craving, and relapse. *Addict. Recovery* **11,** 17–18.

[44]B. C. Wallace (1990c) Treating crack cocaine dependence: the critical role of relapse prevention. *J. Psychoactive Drugs* **22,** 149–158.

[45]T. Todd (1989) Treatment of crack and cocaine abusers. Paper presented at the conferences, "What Works: An International Perspective on Drug Abuse Treatment and Prevention Research," October 22–25, 1989, New York.

[46]G. A. Marlatt (1988) Matching client to treatment: Treatment models and stages of change, in *Assessment of Addictive Behaviors.* D. M. Donovan and G. A. Marlatt, eds. Guilford, New York.

[47]F. Schiffer (1988) Psychotherapy of nine successfully treated cocaine abusers: Techniques and Dynamics. *J. Subst. Abuse Treatment* **5,** 131–137.

[48]A. T. McLellan (1986) "Psychiatric severity" as a predictor of outcome from substance abuse treatments, in *Psychopathology and Addictive Disorders.* R. E. Meyers, ed. Guilford, New York.

Index

M

N

O

P

R

S

T